MASTERING
CONCEPT-BASED TEACHING

A Guide for Nurse Educators

ACG | ACADEMIC CONSULTING GROUP

Elsevier's Academic Consulting Group (ACG) is a coalition of experienced educators and administrators dedicated to helping nursing programs succeed. The ACG provides consulting services and faculty development workshops to help individual institutions plan and implement a concept-based curriculum. ACG consultants can help you:

- Develop a concept based curriculum including selecting concepts and exemplars
- Create objectives, lesson plans and activities for a successful classroom experience
- "Flip" the classroom to maximize student involvement
- Incorporate conceptual teaching into clinical experiences
- Evaluate the impact of a CBC at an individual school

To learn more visit academicconsulting.elsevier.com

MASTERING
CONCEPT-BASED TEACHING

A Guide for Nurse Educators

JEAN FORET GIDDENS, PhD, RN, FAAN
RWJF Executive Nurse Fellow
Dean and Professor
School of Nursing
Virginia Commonwealth University
Richmond, Virginia

LINDA CAPUTI, EdD, MSN, CNE, ANEF
President
Linda Caputi, Inc.
Professor Emerita
College of DuPage
Glen Ellyn, Illinois

BETH RODGERS, PhD, RN, FAAN
Professor
College of Nursing
University of New Mexico
Albuquerque, New Mexico

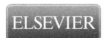

ELSEVIER
MOSBY

3251 Riverport Lane
St. Louis, Missouri 63043

Notices

Knowledge and best practice in this field are constantly changing. As new research and experience broaden our understanding, changes in research methods, professional practices, or medical treatment may become necessary.

Practitioners and researchers must always rely on their own experience and knowledge in evaluating and using any information, methods, compounds, or experiments described herein. In using such information or methods they should be mindful of their own safety and the safety of others, including parties for whom they have a professional responsibility.

With respect to any drug or pharmaceutical products identified, readers are advised to check the most current information provided (i) on procedures featured or (ii) by the manufacturer of each product to be administered, to verify the recommended dose or formula, the method and duration of administration, and contraindications. It is the responsibility of practitioners, relying on their own experience and knowledge of their patients, to make diagnoses, to determine dosages and the best treatment for each individual patient, and to take all appropriate safety precautions.

To the fullest extent of the law, neither the Publisher nor the authors, contributors, or editors, assume any liability for any injury and/or damage to persons or property as a matter of products liability, negligence or otherwise, or from any use or operation of any methods, products, instructions, or ideas contained in the material herein.

Director, Course Solutions: Robin R. Carter
Content Strategist: Lynne Gery
Content Development Specialist: Shephali Graf
Publishing Services Manager: Deborah L. Vogel
Project Manager: Pat Costigan
Design Direction: Karen Pauls
Designer: Renee Duenow

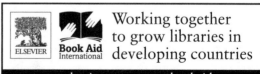

Working together to grow libraries in developing countries

www.elsevier.com • www.bookaid.org

About the Authors

Jean Giddens

Dr. Giddens earned a Bachelor of Science in Nursing from the University of Kansas, a Master of Science of Nursing from the University of Texas at El Paso, and a PhD in Education and Human Resource Studies from Colorado State University. Dr. Giddens has more than 25 years' experience in associate degree, baccalaureate degree, and graduate degree nursing programs in New Mexico, Texas, Colorado, and Virginia. She is an expert in concept-based curriculum and evaluation as well as innovative strategies for teaching and learning. Dr. Giddens serves as an education consultant to nursing programs throughout the country and is the author of multiple journal articles, electronic media, and nursing textbooks, including *Concepts for Nursing Practice.*

Linda Caputi

Dr. Caputi earned an MSN from Loyola University, Chicago, and an EdD from Northern Illinois University. She is a Certified Nurse Educator and a fellow in the NLN's Academy of Nursing Education. Dr. Caputi is Professor Emeritus, College of DuPage. She has won six awards for teaching excellence from Sigma Theta Tau and has been included for three years in *Who's Who Among America's Teachers.* She is the author or editor of five books, chapter contributor for six books, and has published many journal articles, all on nursing education. Dr. Caputi is President of Linda Caputi, Inc., a nursing education consulting company, and she has worked with hundreds of nursing programs on topics related to revising curriculum, transforming clinical education, and numerous other nursing education topics.

Beth Rodgers

Dr. Rodgers earned a Bachelor of Science degree in Nursing from Georgia State University and an MSN and PhD in Nursing from the University of Virginia. She has devoted more than 28 years to nursing education at the undergraduate and graduate levels and to research to expand knowledge about the experiences of people living with chronic conditions. She is recognized widely for her expertise in nursing as a discipline and the development of nursing knowledge, and Dr. Rodgers is frequently sought as a consultant in nursing epistemology, as well as concept and theory development in doctoral education in nursing. She is the author or editor of two popular textbooks on knowledge and concept development, along with an extensive array of book chapters and journal articles.

Preface

The education reform movement over the past two decades has been propelled by an expansion in what we know related to human learning. Advances in brain research related to the process of thinking and learning have had a significant influence on the practice of teaching. Research has shown that learning is influenced by the ability to make connections between information and that such connections form knowledge structures that facilitate the application of information to multiple situations. This process is at the heart of the *conceptual approach*. Thus, the science of learning has led to the rise of the conceptual approach in primary and secondary education as well as higher education. In recent years, significant interest in the conceptual approach has grown in nursing education. This increased interest parallels the education discipline and is seen as a way to manage excessive curriculum content through information management, to engage students, to develop the thinking skills of nursing students, and to produce highly skilled nursing graduates who can manage patients in an increasingly complex health care system.

The conceptual approach represents the incorporation of concepts, exemplars, concept-based curriculum, concept-based instruction, and conceptual learning into the practice of nurse educators. For most faculty, the conceptual approach represents a considerable change in the way the curriculum is structured and taught. It requires a collective reframing of the education process among faculty and students. Although there is significant interest in adopting the conceptual approach in nursing programs, many faculty groups have not had adequate exposure to this approach or clear guidance and therefore lack the expertise or understanding. They may have teaching expertise but just not in conceptual teaching, which is needed for optimal success.

This book was written specifically as a resource for the conceptual approach in nursing education. Targeted users of this book include nursing faculty in undergraduate or graduate nursing programs and graduate nursing students who are preparing for a career in academia. This book does not attempt to replicate the many excellent resources that exist related to general education on faculty roles, teaching strategies, and curriculum development. However, this book does present these topics within the context of the conceptual approach. It is also not expected that an individual will read this book sequentially from cover to cover—so each chapter stands alone and is beneficial in relation to the desired topic area.

- Chapter 1 focuses on the conceptual approach as a general overview. It is an excellent starting point for faculty who want a broad "30,000-foot" view of the conceptual approach and the various elements.
- Chapters 2 and 3 provide a deep look into concepts and understanding what is meant by concept analysis; these chapters are presented from a theoretical lens and are intended to deepen the understanding of concepts; this understanding is foundational to the conceptual approach.
- Chapter 4 provides a discussion about how to develop a concept-based curriculum. Although this process mirrors any other curriculum development process, concepts are used as the infrastructure for the curriculum, and this chapter explains how.
- Chapter 5 offers readers a look into what is now known about how the human brain works, and it demonstrates how the use of concepts enhances learning.
- Chapter 6 presents a discussion of conceptual teaching and how this differs from traditional content-focused instruction. Furthermore, the reader is provided examples of specific teaching strategies that result in conceptual learning.
- Chapter 7 delivers an overview of evaluation strategies that faculty can use to determine achievement of student learning—again with a specific emphasis on conceptual learning.

Important to note, the seven chapters in this book are closely interrelated to one another—in other words, some overlap is unavoidable. For example, part of the development and implementation of a concept-based curriculum (Chapter 4) includes the development of teaching strategies (Chapter 6) and the curriculum evaluation plan (Chapter 7). As another example, the development of effective teaching strategies (Chapter 6) requires the foundational understanding of concepts (Chapters 2 and 3) and an understanding of human learning with concepts (Chapter 5).

This book represents the collaborative efforts of three experienced nurse educators with the intent of harnessing their wide and varied expertise into a useful resource for our faculty colleagues who are courageous enough to embark on the conceptual approach journey. We hope this book will serve you well along the way!

Jean Giddens
Linda Caputi
Beth Rodgers

Foreword

How we think about creating learning opportunities has changed. Teachers are heartily rejecting the notion of content saturation as a satisfactory method and philosophy for teaching. The time has come for a relevant, focused resource that helps those who teach, "***create the compelling learning environment***" that Carol Tomlinson speaks of in the Erickson foreword above. Our goals for teaching must simply move beyond the axiom of "covering the content." Instead, our students' experiences with learning should be satisfying and successful. Concept-based learning is today's hope that this could actually occur.

It is especially fortunate that the "first team" is authoring this resource. Each of the authors—Jean Giddens, Linda Caputi, and Beth Rodgers—is a nursing education pioneer in her own right. How helpful to have the perspectives of all three experts converge as they think about the theory and application of *how to do* concept-based learning.

Our own foray into concept-based learning at the University of Kansas started in 2009, when we realized that our 15-year-old BSN curriculum was tired and outdated. Discerningly, and skeptically, our faculty carefully considered a number of options before deciding on a concept-based learning approach. Frankly, we floundered without adequate resources—and though our end result is quite good, we truly would have benefitted from a complete, coherent, faculty-oriented introduction to the topic.

That introduction is now in your hands—or on your computer. And, happily, in it you will find what you need.

The book begins by answering an important question: "Can someone please explain concept-based learning in a way that I can understand?" The authors then provide the thinking and resources to help faculty determine how their schools will identify and develop concepts, and in turn how those concepts are woven together into a coherent curriculum. Whether your faculty works as a committee of the whole or with specific curriculum revision committees—these materials will be very useful to you.

Two important and innovative sections of the book—evidence on brain-based learning, and a contemporary view of evaluation—round out the contributions, giving faculty an up-to-date view of topics critical to understand today's learning landscape.

For faculty development, summer reading, or intensive workshops, this resource will help faculty as they embrace new ways to create a compelling, satisfying and successful learning experience for students. Thank you, authors—for providing what faculty need!

Best wishes,
Nelda Godfrey, PhD, ACNS-BC, FAAN
Associate Dean for Undergraduate Programs
Clinical Professor
University of Kansas School of Nursing
Kansas City, Kansas
March 27, 2014

Acknowledgments

It has been my honor and privilege to work with my two colleagues, Linda Caputi and Beth Rodgers, on this book. Their extraordinary expertise has led to a deepening of my own conceptual understandings. I also extend my gratitude and appreciation to our colleagues at Elsevier, Robin Carter, a long-time friend and advocate, and Shephali Graf who helped us stay on schedule and navigated our work through production. Lastly, I extend my sincere gratitude to our nursing faculty colleagues for moving our profession forward. May the torch burn long and bright!

JFG

Contents

MASTERING
CONCEPT-BASED TEACHING

A Guide for Nurse Educators

The Conceptual Approach—Background and Benefits

Jean Giddens

I f you have been a nurse educator anytime during the past decade, you have likely heard the buzz about the conceptual approach as a basis for curriculum design and teaching. Perhaps you heard about this approach at a conference or from a colleague or read about it in a journal article. Perhaps one or more faculty members from your nursing program have discussed the possibility of adopting a concept-based curriculum as part of a curriculum redesign. Perhaps you are part of a faculty group that is actively developing or implementing a concept-based curriculum. Regardless of how or where you have heard about it, the conceptual approach has been a recent and important trend in nursing education, and its use has been growing exponentially.

You may be wondering what all the buzz is about. Is the conceptual approach merely a gimmicky trend that will pass, or is it part of a transformation of nursing education that is desperately needed? Indeed, educators should be careful not to jump on every bandwagon that comes along. In many cases, education innovations gain immediate interest but are quickly abandoned when implementation proves challenging and or when outcomes fall short of expectations. Most nurse educators have very full workloads and must make the best use of their time. Thus, with regard to any trend, educators are encouraged to consider what is reasonable and not reasonable and what is supported by education science.

A conceptual approach in nursing education may be adopted for many reasons. Among the most important reasons are to manage excessive curriculum content through information management, engage students, develop the thinking skills of nursing students, and produce nursing graduates who are highly skilled in the management of patients in a health care system that is increasingly complex. Successful adoption and implementation of the conceptual approach requires nurse educators to transform the learning environment from the traditional teacher-focused delivery of information to a student-centered environment in which students are actively engaged in the learning process. Carrieri-Kohlman, Lindsey, and West (2003) describe the conceptual approach as "a process that deliberately attempts to examine the nature and substance of nursing from a conceptual perspective" (p. 1). For most nursing programs, the conceptual approach represents a cultural shift in the way faculty and students perceive their roles in the teaching-learning process. The purpose of this chapter is to provide historic background regarding concept-based approaches in education and nursing, describe what is meant by the *conceptual approach*, and present benefits of the conceptual approach for contemporary nursing education.

Background

Many nurse educators might be surprised to learn that the conceptual approach is not a new trend but rather has been borrowed from another discipline and adapted to nursing. Two interesting historical perspectives are associated with the conceptual approach, one from the education discipline and the other from nursing.

The Early Years

In the education discipline, curriculum was historically approached by discrete areas and topical organizers for content, with student learning focused on memorization of facts and practice of discrete skills. As early as the 1950s, Hilda Taba, a visionary educator from San Francisco, proposed the notion of concepts as opposed to topics as content organizers. In her work, concepts are referred to as high-level abstractions; a person's understanding of a concept expands with increasingly complex examples (Taba, 1966). Critics of Taba's work raised concerns about the abstract nature of concepts. It was recognized that unless concepts were clearly defined, they were challenging for faculty to teach in a clear and efficient way.

During this same general period in nursing, many grand theories were emerging, such as those put forth by Dorothea Orem, Sister Callista Roy, and Martha Rogers (Marriner-Tomy & Alligood, 2006). The era of grand theories was a reflection of nursing as a maturing discipline. Grand theories provided a mechanism for the nursing profession to clearly establish itself as a unique and separate health care discipline. Defining professional identity is important work for any profession on its continuum of ongoing development. Subsequently, in the 1970s and 1980s, the design of nursing curricula based on a grand theory became common practice. Because concepts associated with the chosen theory were often used as the foundation for the curriculum, many of these curricula were referred to as "concept based." For example, Orem's Self-Care Framework (Orem, 1971) was widely used as a basis for curriculum development. Orem's theory included the following concepts:

- Self-care
- Self-care agency

- Therapeutic self-care demand
- Self-care deficit
- Nursing agency
- Nursing system

These concepts serve as the building blocks of Orem's theory and are very useful in that context. However, use of these as foundational concepts for a nursing curriculum was problematic for many nursing programs when faculty did not clearly understand the concepts and did not know how to teach conceptually and/or how to link specific content to the concepts. Although nursing faculty in some schools were successful with this type of curriculum design, many educators struggled to translate abstract theoretical concepts to practical application, particularly when teaching novice learners. Interestingly, some of these same issues were experienced within the education discipline.

Education Reform

It was not until the 1990s that significant education reform propelled the idea of different models of curricula and different approaches to teaching. In a study of science and mathematics education, authors described curricula in the United States as "an inch deep and a mile wide" (Schmidt, McKnight, & Raizen, 1997). It became increasingly obvious to educators that the massive content covered in education was limiting true cognitive development (Erikson, 2002). At the same time, increased attention was being directed at research into human learning. In the late 1990s, the National Research Council conducted a study that led to the publication of *How People Learn* (Bransford, Brown, & Cocking, 2000), which provided a synthesis on the science of learning. Bransford and colleagues noted a convergence of evidence across many disciplines with significant implications for education. Advances in brain research related to the process of thinking and learning have influenced teaching, curriculum design, instructional assessment, and learning environments. Thus an emphasis on linking brain research (and the research of learning) to teaching practice has been increasing during the past decade. One of the themes noted from the research is the notion that learning is influenced by students' ability to make connections between information. Even more important, such connections form knowledge structures that allow students to apply knowledge effectively to multiple situations. This process is at the heart of the conceptual approach. Thus the science of learning has influenced the rise of a concept-based curriculum as an alternative to the traditional curriculum models in primary and secondary education (Erikson, 2002, 2008).

Although nursing has been slower to embrace changes in teaching and curriculum design, many nurse educators have taken cues from the education discipline and are becoming increasingly aware of the science supporting new models for teaching and learning, and they are reexamining concept-based approaches. Unlike concept-based curricula of the past (which were largely based on a single grand theory), contemporary concept-based models in nursing education feature common concepts that have emerged from nursing science as the profession has matured. Thus two primary distinctions in present-day concept-based models compared with those of the past are that (1) concepts are less abstract (and easier for faculty and students to understand) and (2) advances in the science of teaching and learning are applied.

The Conceptual Approach

Because many ideas and terms are used to describe the conceptual approach trend in nursing education, clarification is important as a starting point. The term *conceptual approach* in education is broad and represents the incorporation of the following separate but interrelated elements: concepts, exemplars, concept-based curriculum, concept-based instruction, and conceptual learning (Box 1-1). These elements are briefly described here and will be expanded upon in various chapters throughout this text.

Elements of the Conceptual Approach

Concepts

Central to the conceptual approach are concepts. A concept is an organizing idea or mental construct represented by common attributes. In the conceptual approach, concepts form the infrastructure of a concept-based curriculum and are the key elements associated with concept-based instruction and conceptual learning. Concepts represent the key ideas that are used to organize knowledge, facts, skills, and

---

BOX 1-1 Elements of the Conceptual Approach

Concept: An organizing idea or mental image composed of attributes.
Exemplar: A specific topic or an example represented by the concept.
Concept-based Curriculum: A curriculum that is designed by organizing content around key concepts.
Concept-based Instruction: An instructional process featuring student-centered learning activities that focuses on concepts and the application of information to concepts.
Conceptual Learning: A process by which learners develop high-level thinking skills and the ability to apply facts in the context of related concepts.

competencies across multiple situations and contexts. Concepts function as hubs for transferable knowledge.

Any given discipline, including nursing, contains an endless number of concepts that range from the very broad (known as *macroconcepts*) to the narrow (known as *microconcepts*). Several concepts can link to each macroconcept, and several microconcepts can link to each concept (Figure 1-1). A critical task of educators who adopt the conceptual approach is to identify and clearly address the key concepts to be used. Not only should concepts be selected on the basis of relevancy to the discipline and the program of study, but they also should be organized logically within the curriculum and be used consistently by faculty for maximum benefit to the learner. Achieving such consistency among faculty requires a solid understanding (and agreement) of how the concepts are to be used in the curriculum across courses, how to present the concepts in a useful way to students, and how to link essential content knowledge to the concepts for in-depth understanding. Additionally, faculty must help students recognize

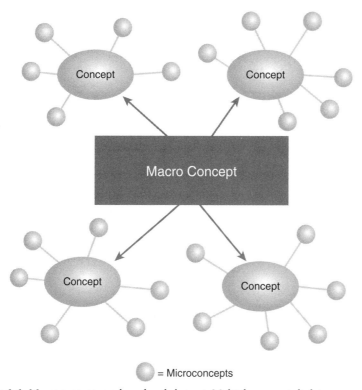

= Microconcepts

Figure 1-1 Macroconcepts are broad and abstract. Multiple concepts link to a macroconcept. Microconcepts are narrow, specific, and tend to be associated with specialty practice/knowledge.

the relationships among the key concepts, because in most clinical situations several concepts are involved (which are referred to as *interrelated concepts*). For example, Figure 1-2 shows the concept *Health Promotion* and several key interrelated concepts. In this example, three different concept categories are represented: *Health and Illness* (at the right), *Professional Nursing* (at bottom, left), and *Patient Attribute* (top). Each of these interrelated concepts not only link to health promotion but also link to each other (as illustrated by the arrows). Interrelated concept diagrams help visualize the interrelationships and illustrate the complexity of concepts. Concepts are discussed in greater detail in Chapters 2 and 3.

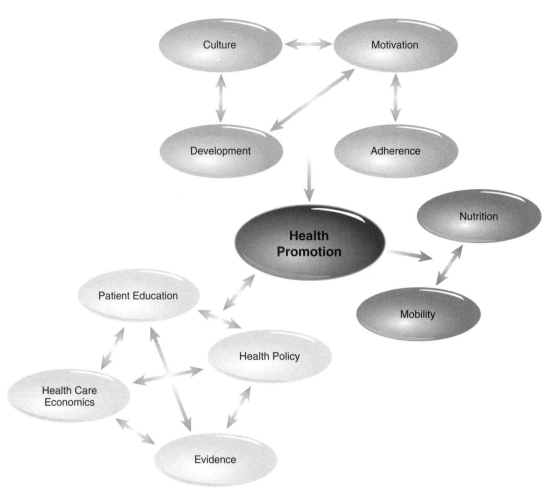

Figure 1-2 Health promotion and interrelated concepts. Interrelationships between attribute concepts, health and illness concepts, and professional nursing concepts. (From Giddens, J. [2013]. *Concepts for nursing practice.* St. Louis, MO: Elsevier.)

Exemplars

Exemplars represent specific topics or content related to a concept. Typically there are many exemplars for any given concept, and exemplars usually connect to multiple concepts. Exemplars are a very important component of the conceptual approach because they represent essential content knowledge. Exemplars provide specific context and help students grasp a deep understanding of the concept. In nursing, exemplars can be health-related conditions experienced by patients (such as asthma, a hip fracture, or an allergic reaction); situations experienced by patients and families in the context of health (such as death and dying, caregiver roles, developmental delays, and bullying); or situations experienced by nurses in the context of professional nursing practice (such as informed consent, use of restraints, medication teaching, and quality improvement projects).

One of the critical tasks of nurse educators who are adopting the conceptual approach is to identify the exemplars to be used for each concept. Faculty members often feel compelled to include multiple exemplars for each concept (usually content from their own specialty or content they have traditionally taught) because of their belief that the content is critical and that students must know it. However, one of the benefits of the conceptual approach is information management, and thus the exemplars should be limited to those most representative or important in helping students attain a grasp of the concept. The learning emphasis should be on the development of cognitive connections. Because exemplars typically link to multiple concepts, faculty should incorporate exemplars in the curriculum plan in such a way that repetitious use of a particular exemplar is avoided. For example, pneumonia could be used effectively as an exemplar for the concepts of gas exchange, infection, acid-base balance, or fatigue. However, it would be unwise to use pneumonia as an exemplar four times within the curriculum, especially considering the many other key content areas that students need to learn. Faculty must help students make purposeful cognitive connections from the exemplar to the primary concept and to other key interrelated concepts. This step is critical to avoid information overload.

A Concept-Based Curriculum

A third element of the conceptual approach is a concept-based curriculum, in which concepts serve as "foundational organizers" that provide an infrastructure to the curriculum. A concept-based curriculum represents a major paradigm shift for nursing because it moves away from an emphasis on content and toward an emphasis on concepts and conceptual learning (Giddens & Brady, 2007). Featured concepts within the courses serve as cornerstones for concept-based instruction and conceptual learning (Giddens et al., 2008). Lynn Erikson, a leading expert in concept-based curriculum and instruction, describes the differences between content-focused and concept-focused curricula as "the difference between memorizing facts related to the American Revolution and developing and sharing ideas related to the concepts of freedom and independence as a result of studying the American Revolution" (Erikson, 2002, p. 50).

When a concept-based curriculum is designed, several key decisions must be made. As with any curriculum, faculty should first determine desired program outcomes or competencies. After this initial step, concept categories or an organizing framework should be developed and concepts should be selected. Each concept should be developed so that faculty members gain a shared understanding about what the concept means and what it represents. Exemplars that will be linked to each concept also must be chosen. Exemplar selection should be based on the best examples of the concept and/or the most common situations represented. Next, decisions regarding the type of courses and the arrangement of concepts within courses must be made, followed by the actual development of each course, and the plan for teaching within the course. Curriculum development also includes a general plan for evaluation to ensure that students attain program outcomes or competencies. Implementation issues include faculty development, student orientation, and maintaining the curriculum integrity. These key decisions and issues are summarized in Box 1-2 and are described further in Chapter 4.

Concept-Based Instruction

A fourth element associated with the conceptual approach is concept-based instruction. This instructional process is characterized by student-centered learning activities that focus on *target concepts* (meaning the featured concept for a unit of study) and the application of key exemplars to concepts. It is worth mentioning again that the focus of instruction is on both the concept (such as a concept overview) *and* the specific exemplars linked to that concept. It is also important

---

BOX 1-2 Key Steps and Decisions When Designing a Concept-Based Curriculum

1. Develop program outcomes
2. Develop an organizing framework for concepts
3. Select and develop featured curriculum concepts
4. Identify exemplars for each concept
5. Organize concepts and exemplars into courses/course development
6. Develop a program evaluation plan

to note that there is not a single or specific instructional strategy for conceptual teaching. Concept-based instruction incorporates a variety of teaching strategies and learning experiences that require higher levels of thinking from faculty and students (Erikson, 2008). Ideally, students are placed in learning groups and work through cases, situations, questions, or problems posed by the instructor as opposed to faculty-centered lectures on concepts. Chapter 6 is devoted to concept-based instructional strategies that support conceptual learning.

Conceptual Learning

Conceptual learning is an active process that engages students. During the learning process, students link factual information and exemplars to concepts. The desired learning outcome is an in-depth understanding of the concept and the ability to transfer ideas to other situations through cognitive connections. Timpson and Bendel-Simso (1996) described conceptual learning as a process through which students learn to organize information into logical mental structures and become increasingly skilled at thinking. In nursing, learning experiences ideally should be placed in the context of a clinical situation and should be purposeful; in other words, learners should clearly recognize the benefit of what they are learning as it pertains to the practice of nursing. Engagement in learning is enhanced when students perceive learning as purposeful and they can see a direct application to their area of study (Ambrose, Bridges, DiPietro, Lovette, & Norman, 2010; Bransford, 2000; Sousa, 2010). Conceptual learning is presented in greater depth in Chapter 5.

 Misconceptions and Clarifications

Misconception: The conceptual approach occurs as a result of designing and implementing a concept-based curriculum.

Clarification: The conceptual approach is attained with the adoption of a concept based curriculum (using concepts and exemplars) and the practice of concept-based instruction to optimize conceptual learning.

Cohesiveness of the Elements

The Greek philosopher Aristotle is credited with coining the phrase, "The whole is greater than the sum of its parts." This phrase captures the significance of the conceptual approach as a cohesive, comprehensive plan as opposed to a loose collection of one or more elements. The conceptual approach requires a purposeful and planned process whereby concepts influence curriculum design, teaching, and learning. This distinction is important because the incorporation of all five elements (see Box 1-1) is necessary for a successful concept-based educational platform. Although each element stands on its own, a powerful synergistic effect occurs when all the elements are meaningfully incorporated into an education plan. Successful adoption of the conceptual approach in nursing requires a commitment among faculty to follow a concept-based curriculum and to learn how to teach conceptually through carefully designed instructional strategies. Students should be actively engaged in the learning process by applying content in purposeful ways and by learning to make cognitive connections to concepts. The end goal is for learners to gain a deep understanding of the concept and acquire the ability to transfer ideas to other concepts and contexts. This outcome represents the higher-level thinking skills necessary for sound clinical judgment in patient care settings.

Consider the following two scenarios:

Scenario 1

Faculty members of an undergraduate nursing program work very hard to develop a concept-based curriculum. As part of this process, they write learning outcomes, identify key nursing concepts from the literature, agree on exemplars, and develop courses around the concepts. Although some of the faculty members attempt to incorporate more student-centered learning activities in their approach to teaching, the majority continue to use the traditional lecture format and focus primarily on exemplars with little to no linkage to the concepts. Additionally, several faculty members become concerned about the loss of what they consider to be "essential information" and add content back into their courses.

Scenario 2

Janice teaches a nursing skills lab in a nursing program that has not undergone a significant curriculum revision in 15 years. After attending a conference presentation on conceptual teaching and learning, Janice decides to adopt a concept-based instructional approach for her course. She identifies key concepts for each unit and uses concept-based teaching strategies to help students link their course content and skills to concepts within her course. Students enrolled in Janice's course find that her teaching strategies are different from those of other faculty. Although most students like the way the course is taught, some students become angry because Janice does not just give them the information they need for the course examinations.

In the first scenario, faculty undoubtedly spent significant time and energy to redesign the curriculum and are proud to have a concept-based curriculum.

However, two primary elements associated with the conceptual approach are missing: a lack of commitment among faculty to adopt concept-based instruction, and a lost opportunity for students to benefit from a conceptual learning experience. The fact that some faculty members elected to add additional content into their courses further undermines the benefit of adopting a concept-based curriculum.

In the second scenario, Janice is motivated to change her teaching methods. By incorporating student-centered learning activities into her instructional method, Janice is becoming increasingly comfortable with and skilled in concept-based instruction. She is also providing an engaging learning environment that is enjoyed by most students in her course. However, because no mechanism is in place for students to encounter the concepts in other courses within the curriculum, the experience occurs in isolation with limited effect.

Although the specific situation in each scenario is different, both scenarios are similar in that one or more elements of the conceptual approach were adopted. However, long-term benefits are unlikely to be achieved because one or more key elements of the conceptual approach were not incorporated. Does this mean that complete consensus must be achieved among faculty before they adopt the conceptual approach for their nursing programs? Absolutely not! Gaining complete consensus among any faculty group is unrealistic because of the very nature of academe. A diversity of perspectives, opinions, and values is expected in all organizations. However, for successful adoption of the conceptual approach, critical mass is needed; in other words, adequate support must exist among faculty who teach in the program, and support from the administrative leadership is also necessary.

Benefits of the Conceptual Approach

We are in the midst of widespread change regarding what is known about human learning. What started as a trickle effect has become a force that is changing the landscape of education. The education of students in all disciplines—including nursing—is being dramatically influenced by these events. The conceptual approach links well with this change and offers multiple known benefits, which include addressing content saturation and information management and preparing nurses to successfully practice in complex health care environments by developing conceptual thinking skills that lead to good clinical judgment and collaboration.

Content Saturation

Most educators agree that one of their greatest challenges is having sufficient time to teach all the curriculum content. Although concerns about excessive curriculum content have appeared in the nursing literature for over 30 years, increased attention has been directed at this issue during the past decade (Diekelmann, 2002; Forbes & Hickey, 2009; Giddens & Brady, 2007; Ironside, 2004; National League for Nursing, 2003). Excessive content can be partly attributable to what has been known as the "information age." The exponential generation of new information makes it impossible not only to teach everything that is known in a given discipline but also to keep up with advances and changes in what was previously known. It has been estimated that as much as 50% of the information learned in a 4-year degree program changes within 2 years after graduation. This issue is exacerbated by the traditional "instructor-centric" approach to teaching. Faculty who subscribe to this perspective believe they must "cover" all the content, and the common belief is that students cannot be expected to know anything unless it has been specifically taught in a course. This expectation is quite a burden for any faculty member to carry! With this perspective, classroom time typically becomes little more than information delivery sessions as opposed to learning sessions. Excessive curriculum content has also coincided with the increased size of nursing textbooks (because of the increased generation of nursing knowledge). Many faculty feel obligated to cover large amounts of the information found in textbooks rather than encouraging students to use these books as a learning resource and reference. It is easy to see how the cycle perpetuates the problem. The conceptual approach alleviates the issue of content saturation by limiting the number of concepts and exemplars used and by emphasizing students' ability to make linkages to content to which they are exposed, even if it has not been through formal learning activities within the curriculum. The adage "less is more" applies here, not only in terms of the delivery of content, but more importantly, in the result of better learning.

Information Management

A curriculum focused on content generally emphasizes student memorization of facts (as they are known at that point in time) and does little to prepare students to manage the large volume of changing information they will encounter not only as students but throughout their career. Information management refers to the ability to *locate, analyze, interpret*, and *apply* new information to specific situations. Because it is impossible for any health care professional to know all the information needed to care for all patients, health care professionals must be highly skilled in information management as a basis for evidence-based care. Nursing education must shift from information delivery to the creation of learning environments in which students are required to locate, analyze, interpret, and apply information as part of learning within classroom, laboratory, and clinical environments. These elements are also foundational to conceptual learning. The conceptual approach fosters students' development of information management by learning to link new

---

BOX 1-3 **Exemplar: Information Management in Practice**

Terrin, a nurse working in an inpatient unit, has an order to administer a new pharmacologic agent with which he is unfamiliar. He is told that the agent has only been available for use for 6 months. Terrin logs onto the hospital Intranet website (***locate***) to review the drug information and administration guidelines. Terrin carefully reads the drug information and notices that there are two indications for using the agent; he also notes that the administration guidelines are dependent upon many variables, including intended use, age, weight, and underlying medical conditions (***analyze***). Based on the information presented, Terrin gains an understanding regarding the specific context for which the agent was ordered (***interpret***). He uses this information to administer the agent correctly and to monitor the patient for potential adverse effects (***apply***).

---

and emerging information to concept-structures. These elements are described in the following sections, and an example is provided in Box 1-3.

Locate Information

Health care professionals must know how and where to efficiently locate accurate information on which to base their practice. More specifically, this ability means knowing appropriate and reliable sources (for example, practice, policy, or procedure guidelines and evidence-based practice findings) and having the skill to access these sources (such as through the Internet, Intranet, or a resource manual).

Analyze Information

Analysis of information requires a critical examination of information elements to determine the relationship of the parts or to discover meaning. New information and the supporting evidence are often complex, requiring careful consideration of all elements. Health care professionals must be able to gain an accurate understanding of new information through analysis of the information that is available.

Interpret Information

The process of information analysis should lead to the ability of the health care professional to draw meaning from the information. One aspect of the process is to analyze the information, but a key component is the ability to translate the information into understandable terms or context. The process of interpretation means gaining an understanding of the meaning or significance of the information. In the context of health care, this process means gaining an understanding of how the information fits with the context of care within the clinical environment.

Apply Information

The evidence-based practice movement ultimately is about applying the latest evidence or information to one's practice. Application of information refers to the process of putting newly learned or discovered information to use. It is assumed that the newly discovered/learned information comes from a reliable source. In the context of health care, the information must be applied correctly to provide evidence-based care.

Student Learning and Engagement

Another significant benefit of the conceptual approach is the emphasis on student learning as opposed to the instruction provided by faculty. By and large, the emphasis in education has been on what the instructor does; this notion is captured very well by Bellack, who noted that "…nursing education continues to be 'teaching heavy' and 'learning light'" (Bellack, 2008, p. 439). With the conceptual approach, learning occurs when students develop skills in building cognitive connections to previous learning as opposed to learning facts. The end result is that learners become more effective and efficient thinkers and problem solvers.

Collaboration

Effective, coordinated health care delivery depends on collaboration among health care professionals. Teamwork and Collaboration, one of the six core competencies from Quality & Safety Education for Nurses (QSEN), emphasizes the need for nurses to be skilled collaborators, not only with other nurses but also with persons from other disciplines (QSEN, 2013). Teams and Teamwork is also a core competency identified by the Interprofessional Education Collaborative (IPEC) Expert Panel (IPEC, 2011). Thus there is little doubt that graduates of nursing programs need a strong foundation in collaboration. Collaborative learning is at the heart of the conceptual approach. Historically, higher education has rewarded individual achievement, and this perspective is reinforced in a traditional classroom, where students take in information and are tested on the content. The conceptual approach requires students to learn in groups, and thus collaborative learning in school translates well to collaboration in clinical practice. If nurse educators are sincere in setting expectations that nursing graduates "play well with others," then collaborative learning must occur as a part of the education process from the first to last semesters.

In addition to facilitating collaborative learning, the conceptual approach also provides a platform to design interprofessional learning activities, events, and courses. Most concepts found in a nursing curriculum actually apply to all health care disciplines. For example, students enrolled in medicine, nursing, pharmacy, dentistry, or physical therapy all must learn about concepts such as *Culture, Ethics, Health Promotion, Informatics, Quality, Safety, Infection,* and *Gas Exchange.* Despite the fact that many of these concepts have universal application, each discipline plays a unique role in the provision of health care as it relates to the concepts. The conceptual approach provides a unique opportunity for the development of a robust core interprofessional curriculum featuring collaborative learning and team-based care across disciplines.

From Conceptual Thinking to Clinical Judgment

Nursing graduates must develop skill in clinical reasoning and clinical judgment for success in an increasingly complex health care environment. The linear approach to learning in traditional content-focused curricula does little to facilitate skills needed by nurses in the complex health care system. Tanner's model of clinical judgment (Tanner, 2006) illustrates that a nurse's response to a clinical situation is influenced by his or her previous experiences with regard to a situation, noticing when patterns are inconsistent with a given situation (i.e., taking into consideration the context of the situation), and correctly interpreting and clarifying information (Figure 1-3). The development of conceptual thinking skills facilitates clinical reasoning because of the cognitive connections to concepts made by students when

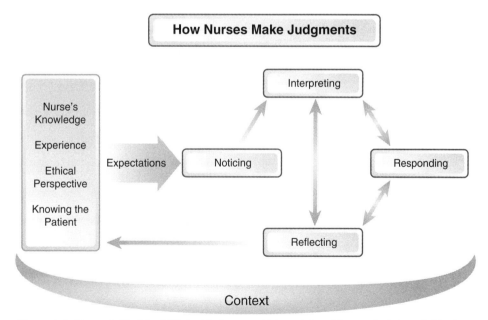

Figure 1-3 Tanner's Model of Clinical Judgment. (Adapted from Tanner, C. A. [2006]. Thinking like a nurse: A research-based model of clinical judgment in nursing. *Journal of Nursing Education, 45*[60], 204–211.)

encountering new information. Having an in-depth understanding of a concept provides the necessary platform for students and practicing nurses.

Summary

As the health care environment becomes increasingly complex, nursing programs need to respond by preparing graduates to manage information effectively, provide patient-centered care that is evidence based, and work well within teams. These goals will require a transformation of nursing education curricula and teaching practices from an instructor-centered and content-focused paradigm to the conceptual approach. This chapter introduces the conceptual approach, reinforcing the notion that five key elements—concepts, exemplars, concept-based curriculum, concept-based instruction, and conceptual learning—must be in place for optimal success (see Box 1-1). Benefits of the conceptual approach include addressing content saturation, information management, enhanced student learning and engagement, collaboration, and supporting the development of clinical judgment. In the chapters that follow, key elements and processes are presented in greater detail to enhance understanding and application in teaching practice.

REFERENCES

Ambrose SA, Bridges MW, DiPietro M, Lovette MC, Norman MK: *How learning works. 7 research-based principles for smart teaching*, San Francisco, CA, 2010, Jossey-Bass.

Bellack J: Letting go of the rock, *Journal of Nursing Education* 47(10):439–440, 2008.

Bransford JD, Brown AL, Cocking RR: *How people learn: Brain, mind, experience, and school*, Washington, DC, 2000, National Academy Press.

Carrieri-Kohlman V, Lindsey AM, West CM: *Pathophysiological phenomena in nursing: Human response to illness*, ed 3, Philadelphia, PA, 2003, Saunders.

Diekelmann N: "Too much content…." Epistemologies' grasp and nursing education, *Journal of Nursing Education* 41(11):469–470, 2002.

Erikson L: *Concept-based curriculum and instruction*, Thousand Oaks, CA, 2002, Corwin Press.

Erikson L: *Stirring the head, heart, and soul. Redefining curriculum, instruction, and concept-based learning*, Thousand Oaks, CA, 2008, Corwin Press.

Forbes MO, Hickey MT: Curriculum reform in baccalaureate nursing education: Review of the literature, *International Journal of Nursing Education Scholarship* 6(1), Article 27, 2009.

Giddens J, Brady D: Rescuing nursing education from content saturation: The case for a concept-based curriculum, *Journal of Nursing Education* 46(2):65–69, 2007.

Giddens J, Brady D, Brown P, Wright M, Smith D, Harris J: A new curriculum for a new era of nursing education, *Nursing Education Perspectives* 29(4):200–204, 2008.

Interprofessional Education Collaborative Expert Panel: *Core competencies for interprofessional collaborative practice: Report of an expert panel*, Washington, DC, 2011, Interprofessional Education Collaborative.

Ironside PM: "Covering content" and teaching thinking: Deconstructing the additive curriculum, *Journal of Nursing Education* 43(1):5–12, 2004.

Marriner-Tomy A, Alligood MR: *Nursing theorists and their work*, St. Louis, MO, 2006, Elsevier.

National League for Nursing: *Position statement: Innovation in nursing education: A call to reform. 2003*, http://www.nln.org/aboutnln/PositionStatements/innovation.htm

Orem D: *Nursing: Concepts of Practice*, Columbus, OH, 1971, McGraw-Hill.

Quality & Safety Education for Nurses Institute (n.d.) Competencies. http://qsen.org/competencies/

Schmidt WH, McKnight CC, Raizen S: *A splintered vision: An investigation of U.S. Science and mathematics education. U.S. National Research Center for the Third International Mathematics and Science Study (TIMSS)*, Dordrecht, Netherlands, 1997, Kluwer Academic Publishers.

Sousa DA: *Mind, brain, and education. Neuroscience implications for the classroom*, Bloomington, IN, 2010, Solution Tree Press.

Taba H: *Teaching strategies and cognitive functioning in elementary school children. Cooperative research project*, Washington, DC, 1966, Office of Education, U.S. Department of Health, Education, and Welfare.

Tanner CA: Thinking like a nurse: a research-based model of clinical judgment in nursing, *Journal of Nursing Education* 45(6):204–211, 2006.

Timpson WM, Bendel-Simso P: *Concepts and choices for teaching: Meeting the challenges in higher education*, Madison, WI, 1996, Magna Publications.

Concepts in the Discipline of Nursing

2

Beth Rodgers

Concept-based curricula and a concept-focused approach to teaching are not new phenomena, as noted elsewhere in this book. However, the concept-focused approach is likely to be new for many nurse educators who are more accustomed to focusing on content in the form of "facts" or "principles" rather than on broader ideas or concepts. An irony is inherent in the idea that a concept-based approach may be unique, however, because human beings work with concepts all the time and, in fact, much of what nurses do is based on having a good grasp of the concepts critical to nursing practice. Learning is, to a great extent, a process of concept acquisition, and knowledge involves the formation, clarification, and application of concepts. A concept-based curriculum requires that the conceptual foundation for nursing be at the forefront of teaching and learning rather than something that occurs on a more abstract level secondary to the acquisition of principles and data. To assist students in this process, faculty who use this approach need to have a thorough understanding of concepts, including what they are, how they are formed, how they are used in nursing, how they make up the discipline of nursing, and what functions they serve with regard to knowledge in general.

An Overview of Concepts in Nursing Education

On a general level, a concept-based approach to teaching helps put a focus on knowing rather than doing. Nurses are strikingly adept at answering questions about what nursing is with an emphasis on what they are able to do or what tasks they perform in the course of their work. When an individual nurse is asked, "What is it like to be a nurse?" a common response often is, "Well, I work in (setting) and do…." The response may even include a reference to the ubiquitous "caring," a gerund that sometimes implies action and tasks. A focus on concepts and conceptual learning makes it possible to take the knowledge that the nurse possesses and look at it in the abstract, outside of an immediate application, initially, thus helping to recognize that there is thought and cognitive power in the concept. That thought or knowledge then can be applied to nursing situations that include patient care or other health-related foci. A nurse with a strong conceptual grasp of the discipline, instead of describing tasks, would talk about the creation of empathic relationships with care recipients, whether they be individuals, families, or communities. A nurse who works with persons who have chronic heart disease, for example, could describe using concepts such as *Mobility*, *Gas Exchange*, and *Self-Management* to help the patient adjust his or her activities to achieve a level of independence and quality of life that is consistent with individual life goals and physiologic capacities. The nurse also could relay that he or she has a strong grasp of the illness trajectory and the threats to identity that often accompany chronic illness and, rather than focusing primarily on monitoring for medication adherence and physiologic stability or deterioration, works with an understanding of what it is like to live with a chronic condition to help the patient maintain dignity and self-worth. The nurse also would understand the importance of social support in such a situation and work with the patient to develop appropriate strategies to achieve reasonable goals in the situation. Such a description would be quite a change from how a nurse otherwise might describe this type of work, perhaps saying merely, "I work with people who have heart disease."

This approach sometimes is confused with "holism," an important aspect of nursing and one of the characteristics that differentiates it from other disciplines. A holistic focus is not the same as a conceptual focus, however. Holism refers to how the nurse uses the concepts to approach a patient, family, or community health situation. Holism involves the use of multiple concepts to address the many factors and challenges that are present in any encounter. Holism thus provides a perspective or framework for ensuring that multiple concepts are addressed in the situation as appropriate. The concept focus emphasizes the concepts and knowledge that are used to create that holistic approach. A focus on concepts thus is a focus on knowledge first, rather than action. Clearly, knowledge should precede action, and such a focus in the acquisition of cognitive content enables more widespread application than a focus on specific tasks or activities would allow.

A good example of one of the differences in concept-based learning is the concept of *Asepsis*. In a skills-oriented course, the nursing student will learn how to insert an indwelling urinary catheter and all of the appropriate steps in that process. The student also will learn about isolation technique, handwashing, and numerous other physical skills. If the student has a strong grasp of the concept of *Asepsis*, however, he or she can apply that cognitive content across this variety of physical actions. Without the concept of *Asepsis*, the student is in a position of memorizing the steps of each procedure as if they were unrelated. A solid understanding of a concept enables the student (or anyone who grasps the concept) to identify similarities across situations and transfer knowledge from one context to the next.

This example using the concept of *Asepsis* reveals one valuable feature of concepts: They are important organizational elements, providing a way of clustering knowledge that enables someone with a strong grasp of a concept to move from one situation to another with some knowledge that helps that person interpret the new situation. Nurses cannot approach every encounter as a completely unique situation, nor can they manage each interaction as if it were an isolated case study. It is necessary to have some way of grasping information and organizing it so it is available for application across varied encounters. Concepts serve that purpose, making it possible to carry knowledge from one situation to another (Figure 2-1). In applying the concepts, it also becomes clear when the concepts need to be refined or improved to be of greater use. In the case of more abstract concepts, such as *Dignity*, *Quality of Life*, or *Autonomy*, this theoretical power of concepts becomes particularly evident. Knowledge about such important aspects of human existence cannot be obtained by learning how to name something or by pointing

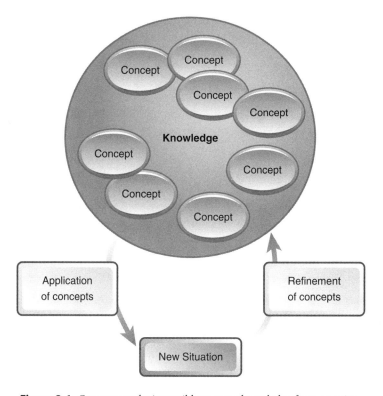

Figure 2-1 Concepts make it possible to carry knowledge from one situation to another and then to refine the concepts.

to an object and saying, "That is *Justice*." No physical objects correspond to such concepts; consequently, clear abstract knowledge is needed even to discuss such things. Concepts serve this purpose in that they are very powerful theoretical clusters of knowledge.

This emphasis on knowledge and the ability to learn and carry information from one situation to the next are key aspects of a concept-based curriculum. To enact such a curriculum and engage in concept-based teaching, it is necessary to have a thorough understanding of what is meant by the term "concept." In other words, the educator, as well as the student, must have a meaningful concept of what a concept is. It is also important to understand how concepts are communicated and shared. Without some way to discuss concepts and share ideas, a concept-based curriculum would not be possible. Language and experience also are important components of an understanding of concepts.

In nursing, concepts have been identified as important elements of knowledge for decades. Much of the work on concepts in nursing historically was focused either on how to make them more clear or on the task of analyzing or synthesizing concepts as a way of developing the knowledge base. Catherine Norris (1982) was one of the first persons to focus on concepts in the context of the nursing knowledge base with her text *Concept Clarification in Nursing*. The work of Walker and Avant (1988, 1995, 2011) is included in many courses oriented toward a discussion of theory in nursing. Along with Norris, Walker and Avant presented nurses with ideas about concept analysis and ushered in a particular focus on analysis that continues decades later. Chinn and Kramer (1991, 2011) also addressed concepts in their writings, particularly with regard to concept development, and it is worth noting that later editions of the popular theory text authored by Meleis (1997, 2012) included a discussion of concepts and the role of concepts in the knowledge base of nursing.

The most common discussions of concepts in nursing since the 1980s, and continuing to the present, have involved the idea of concepts as "building blocks of theory" and, related to that, an emphasis on analysis of concepts (King, 1988). With regard to analysis, a myriad of publications have presented the results of analyses of concepts using diverse approaches and with varying levels of rigor. Although an extensive array of concepts has been addressed in this manner, and multiple analyses have been performed for many concepts, little effort has been expended to tie the analyses to substantive epistemic, scientific, or clinical problems in the discipline. As a result, the literature abounds with articles on concepts and attempts to clarify concepts with minimal connection to how such approaches solve actual problems or enhance the knowledge base of the discipline (Rodgers, 1989, 2000). Because the turn toward concept-based curricula is occurring again, addressing the discussion of concepts in a more substantive manner is imperative.

What Is a Concept?

A thorough discussion of concepts can go in numerous directions, because concepts have many roles in human existence. As noted previously, concepts are major components of knowledge, theoretical constructions, and organizational tools for thinking. They also can be creative elements, ideas or mental images, essential components of communication, and parts of larger theories. All of these foci point not only to the critical nature of concepts in human cognition and learning but also to the many different roles and uses of concepts that need to be considered to develop a clear understanding of what a concept is.

In general, and from a knowledge standpoint, a concept is "an abstraction that is expressed in some form" (Rodgers, 1989, p. 3), which may seem like a rather simple statement to reflect the essential nature of concepts and the many roles that they play in human existence. Yet this idea of being abstract and being linked to some form of expression is at the core of the definition of "concept." In general, concepts are formed through encounters with various situations and phenomena and the ability to see similarities in those encounters. As a result, the mind forms images that include those common characteristics.

 Misconceptions and Clarifications

| **Misconception:** A concept is something that can be seen or directly measured. | **Clarification:** Although some concepts can be represented by a physical object, many concepts do not have a corresponding physical object and are represented by ideas, abstractions, mental images, or other modalities. |

A child learning what is meant by the word "dog" is a simple example of this process. The child might live with a retriever, visit a family that has a terrier, and have a neighbor with a poodle. The child will hear the word "dog" used to refer to those animals. In a short amount of time the child recognizes that these creatures have some things in common and that the word "dog" does not refer to any specific animal but is applicable to an array of animals that have certain characteristics in common. Hearing the word "dog" stimulates a mental image or idea—that is, the concept of *Dog* that has been formed from a composite of those common characteristics. "Pluto" would be an example of a proper name for a specific dog; "dog" is the term used to express an idea of general characteristics common to all dogs. In conversation, someone might say, "I have a dog," and the person to whom he or she is speaking will immediately know something about the animal to which the original speaker is referring even if that animal is not present during the conversation. The concept that is stimulated upon hearing the word "dog" does not specify the type of dog, age, size, or activity level; rather, each individual may have a distinct concept of *Dog* based on experience, familiarity, exposure, and even preference. Still, because each individual in the conversation possesses the concept of *Dog*, with its common characteristics, it is possible to refer to something that is not present, to understand such references, and to understand each other and carry on meaningful communication (Rodgers, 2000).

Concepts also are developed in a person in other ways because not all concepts have physical examples such as *Dog* to facilitate their learning. Concepts such as *Dignity*, *Personhood*, *Grief*, *Health*, *Vulnerability*, and *Resilience* are very important in nursing yet do not have corresponding objects that can be pointed to as examples of these concepts. Such concepts are developed through exposure to ideas, human creativity, storytelling, and other modalities. They also are developed through contact with examples and by having the opportunity to experience situations in which the concept exists, even if those situations are not specifically related to the concept on a one to one basis as is the case with physical objects.

Concepts are acquired in different ways, but as the previous example indicates, socialization can be an important part of the process. If the child is only exposed to small dogs, the concept will be constructed on the basis of that exposure and familiarity. The child who later encounters a Great Dane or mastiff might find that his or her initial concept of *Dog* is challenged and will have to reevaluate, or learn in a new way, that these situations are also appropriate for application of the concept of *Dog*.

A similar socialization process is at work with other types of concepts, and the profound influence of context is evident in numerous examples in nursing. Many of the concepts that are crucial to the work of nurses do have tangible examples to facilitate learning; an example is the concept of *Sphygmomanometer*. When the student has a grasp of that concept, he or she will understand the nature of the sphygmomanometer whether it is an older mercury tube model, an aneroid model, or an electronic variation. Note that the concept of something is not the object itself. Distinctions exist between (1) the *concept* of *Sphygmomanometer*—that is, the mental or cognitive "idea" about such a tool (an implement of various types that is used to measure blood pressure because it can detect the pressure of the blood against the arterial wall), (2) the *object* sphygmomanometer (that sphygmomanometer over there or one that is physically present), and (3) the *term* "sphygmomanometer" (i.e., the word that is used to express the concept). The student will have to learn how to operate the specific model, but upon knowing that it is a sphygmomanometer, he or she will immediately know its use in a patient care situation.

Concepts such as *Dignity*, *Grief*, *Autonomy*, *Quality of Life*, *Safety*, *Patient-centered*, and an abundance of others also are crucial to professional nursing practice, yet no objects exist that can be pointed to as examples of these concepts. In such instances the abstract nature of concepts becomes particularly apparent. These examples also make it is easy to see how socialization, education, and personal experience and values can influence the particular concept that any nurse holds. Cultural differences in the expression of and norms surrounding many of these concepts are documented extensively. *Grief* is a particularly good example of how norms vary in the formation of a concept (Cowles & Rodgers, 2000), and the value and expressions of autonomy vary with age, gender, and other demographic factors. Many other concepts used in nursing and health care are specific to the professionals. *Health Literacy*, for example, is not a concept that the recipients of care generally work with or possess; it is a concept used by the care providers to address an aspect of understanding and involvement in care.

Why Are Concepts Important?

This discussion about concept acquisition, behavior, and language reveals why concepts are important and are an appropriate focal point in education. Concepts are the objects of thought, and they are organizational elements for thinking. Because of common understandings of language, it is possible to communicate our ideas and concepts with others. It is important to acknowledge that although different people might use the same word to describe a situation, it does not mean that they possess the same concept. Nonetheless, without a connection between concepts and some form of expression, typically a formal language, communication is not possible. Similarly, without some connection between concepts and action, behavior and actions become random, isolated, and based on a case or situation, without the ability to apply knowledge across varied instances. The formation of concepts is essential to learning and to learned action, and conversely, part of the purpose of learning is to promote in the learner the development of concepts that are relevant, effective, and of practical use.

Although concepts are, to some extent, "building blocks of theory," a statement that is found widely throughout nursing theory texts, concepts actually are powerful theoretical packages on their own. Without concepts, the mind is merely a mirror reflecting what exists in the world outside of the mind or a scattered conglomerate of ideas and impressions developed in the creative mind. Moving from one encounter or situation to the next would require starting anew, without a knowledge foundation to use when approaching that next situation. Concepts are not merely words but are collections of characteristics abstracted from reality, and they typically contain the values, experiences, and socialization of the person who possesses the concepts, which makes them not only essential components of knowledge but powerful tools for effective action.

Divergent Approaches to Concepts

The previous discussion of concepts was focused on a general overview of what concepts are and how they are linked to language and behavior. Some additional discussion of concepts can be helpful in understanding the importance of some otherwise subtle differences in how concepts are viewed. The educator in a concept-based curriculum needs to have a solid understanding of the nature of concepts and the various aspects of concepts and influences on their development to create appropriate learning experiences and assessments.

A discussion of the nature of concepts can be found throughout a large volume of literature in numerous disciplines. Philosophers have studied and discussed concepts with regard to the study of knowledge (epistemology) and the role that concepts play in the formation of knowledge. In addition to this epistemic focus, philosophers also have explored modes of communication and language (linguistic philosophy), which includes discussion of concepts, and analytic philosophy has been focused on concepts with regard to their relationships to both sentence structure and correspondence with reality. Sociologists have discussed concepts as indicators of societies and group behavior, in addition to the role of concepts and conceptual problems in their own discipline (Lizardo, 2013; Sundbo, 2013), and anthropologists have undertaken similar work in realms related to culture and acculturation. Cognitive psychologists also rely on an understanding of concepts in explanations of learning and knowledge acquisition (Mahon & Caramazza, 2009).

The term "concept" also appears in the literature of other fields with slightly different uses. In the literature of business, references to "concepts" for marketing or product innovation are distinct from the epistemic or knowledge-oriented "concepts" of interest in curriculum development. Yet even this use points to the cognitive or mental aspect of concept formation—that is, creating in the minds of consumers a particular idea about a product and the need for the latest innovation. New products also can lead to new behaviors, as anyone who has witnessed the pre- and post-personal computer era has experienced (Rodgers, 2000). All of these examples indicate that concepts, regardless of focus, constitute an important component of knowledge, learning, socialization, and human existence.

Ambiguity About Concepts

In spite of extensive writing in numerous disciplines, a long history of emphasis on concepts in education, and the recent resurgence of interest in concepts as a focus of teaching, widespread disagreement and considerable vagueness exist concerning a number of details about concepts. Concepts are incredibly powerful and important in the lives of human beings and certainly in the behaviors of the professional nurse. However, in spite of a common general understanding of what concepts are, there is much room for debate about how they are formed in the mind, how shared meanings can develop, how concepts can be taught, what the role of socialization is in the development of individual concepts and collections of concepts, and how the possession or grasp of a particular concept affects behavior and action. In the case of nursing and education, the need to understand how concepts can be taught and how deeper understanding can be developed in students is particularly pressing so the students can acquire the knowledge necessary to perform at a high level. The challenge is much greater than immediate learning, however, because the competent nurse must continue to learn and be willing to change his or her knowledge and behaviors based on changes in knowledge and concepts, and then he or she must demonstrate the application of changes in knowledge through changes in practice. Nurses whose knowledge and actions are limited by context and who are static or unresponsive to new discoveries are not performing in a manner that is consistent with the standards of professional nursing practice.

An additional concern involves determining the concepts that are essential to nursing knowledge and how those concepts delineate nursing as a discipline. If nursing education is going to be based on a conceptual approach, a rich understanding regarding concepts in general is needed, along with agreement on a core of concepts that are essential to characterize nursing as a discipline and to provide a substantive basis for reasoned nursing action. The concepts that are selected as the focus for nursing education send a message to students about the core areas of emphasis in the discipline. How those concepts are organized, the language used to communicate them, and the values that are expressed when a concept is shared with students have a considerable impact not only on the learning that takes place but on the socialization of students to the profession of nursing.

A Deeper Look at Concepts

In nursing, concepts often are discussed with an emphasis on their role in theory development, as noted previously. This idea, although widespread in the literature of nursing, will create problems when developing a concept-based curriculum because it gives the impression that theory is needed to link the concepts together to have a sensible and useful knowledge base. Although the value of theory cannot be disputed, concepts themselves are powerful theoretical packages on their own. They can be combined into constructs or into theories, but even when that step is not taken, they are very powerful elements of knowledge. Consistent with the definition provided earlier that concepts are clusters of characteristics of a phenomenon or experience (Rodgers, 2000), concepts develop through experience—either physical, simulated, or created in the mind—through a process of abstraction from experience. The emphasis on thinking or cognition is common throughout discussions of concepts and is found in the literature of nursing as well, in which authors describe concepts as "mental pictures" or "mental images" (Watson, 1979), words or labels (Diers, 1979; Meleis, 1991), or a combination of these (Hardy, 1974). Each approach has strong implications for concept-based curricula and the teaching and learning of concepts in the discipline. Yet none of these approaches alone is sufficient to explain the role of concepts in the discipline or in human cognition and to provide a foundation for curriculum development and the learning of concepts as part of nursing education. Additional exploration of discussions of concepts in the discipline of philosophy can provide more insight into how concepts function as a component of a discipline's knowledge base.

Philosophical Views of Concepts

In the literature of philosophy, concepts generally are viewed in one of two distinct ways, each of which has significant implications for concept-based curricula in nursing. The two major traditions in the discussion of concepts have become known as the "entity view" and the "dispositional view." Each of these views has a unique philosophical perspective with regard to what concepts are, how they are formed, and what purpose they serve relative to the external world. It is therefore reasonable that each viewpoint would lead to different approaches in the teaching and learning of nursing concepts. Implications for curriculum development and teaching will be discussed after we explore these different philosophical perspectives.

Entity Views of Concepts

In simple terms, positions consistent with an entity view consider concepts to be *things* (entities) and, consistent with most philosophers who espouse such a review, these things are ideas in the mind. Variations of entity views were prevalent in early discussions of concepts that can be found in the literature. Typical of those discussions was attention to concepts as mental objects or images that captured broadly applicable or universal characteristics that are found in the physical world. For example, Aristotle (1947, 1984) discussed concepts as universal essences and gave examples such as *Justice* and *Beauty*; no specific objects can be pointed to about which someone can say, "*that* is 'justice'" or "*there* is 'beauty.'" In other words, justice or beauty cannot be evaluated or determined based on the concept corresponding to a physical object. According to this view, however, some external reference exists against which the concept can be judged—that is, the examples of justice or beauty that exist in the real world. Concepts exist in the mind as objects of thinking according to an entity view, but these concepts relate to examples that can be found in physical reality.

Other prominent philosophers who referred to concepts as ideas include Descartes (1644/1960), Locke (1690/1975), and Kant (1781/1965). Although their discussions of concepts in the mind were considerably different, they all focused on concepts as some component of thought. One implication of this philosophical approach with an emphasis on concepts as being in the mind is that concepts can only be evaluated through some means to get inside the mind to examine these objects of thought. Because that is not possible, these philosophical approaches provide no insight into how to evaluate conceptual learning. In fairness to these philosophers, their focus was on the development of knowledge and the acquisition or ascertainment of truth and not on concept development. Thus a focus of their work and writing was on addressing questions related to the connection between physical reality, the workings of the mind, and the development of knowledge.

In spite of the challenge posed by the apparent need to "get inside the mind" to evaluate the concepts held by a person, entity views did provide a basic answer to the critical question about what a concept is. Throughout entity approaches, concepts are addressed as being composed of attributes that are clustered together to capture characteristics that are common in similar objects or occurrences. This notion of concept persists to the present day and is consistent across most discussions of concepts. What varies is not the answer to what a concept *is* but the many other aspects of concepts, including learning, development, the nature of concepts in the context of a discipline of nursing, and the communication or sharing of concepts.

In the mid twentieth century, the focus of discussions of concepts in philosophy shifted from the contents within the mind to an emphasis on language. Philosophers in this era showed a particular interest in how language functioned, particularly in their desire to construct an ideal language that would correspond with reality. Philosophers of this tradition, including Frege (1952a, 1952b) and Wittgenstein (in his earlier writings, 1921/1981), viewed concepts essentially as words that should behave in a very specific way relative to the rules of language (see Frege's writings for a discussion of concepts as predicates). For some philosophers of this genre, the emphasis on language and on correspondence was so critical that a word was not considered to be meaningful unless it did correspond to some object.

The implications of this approach are easy to see in regard to concepts that relate to physical objects. For example, nurses learn about thermometers as part of their education, and an actual physical object exists that can be held in the nurse's hand and is referred to using the term "thermometer." In this case, the word "thermometer" is the proper name of such an object. There also is the *concept* of *Thermometer* that is not any specific thermometer but is an idea the nurse possesses about any number of similar physical objects. They do not all have to look the same or, if electronic or digital, have the same functions and features; the name "thermometer" also can be applied to digital thermometers, glass thermometers, and aural thermometers, for example. However, the nurse has some knowledge of thermometers by possessing the concept; the concept is a cluster of characteristics, abstracted from the physical objects and representative of all items that can be referred to as "thermometer." Evaluation of an individual's concept can be based on whether he or she can identify related objects successfully (i.e., thermometers), communicate about them, and differentiate thermometers from other devices. Correspondence works, to a certain extent, with an array of physical objects.

While the example concerning the concept of *Thermometer* is straightforward, concepts that are important in nursing (and in life in general) often pertain to nonphysical occurrences, as is the case with the concepts of *Professional* or *Dignity* (or *Justice* and *Beauty*, which were mentioned previously). These concepts share the same origin in being formed on the basis of a cluster of characteristics or attributes. Although there is not a physical object that can be pointed to as "professional," it is evident that examples are encountered through the educational process and by way of role modeling and observation. The nurse, or nursing student, can develop a grasp of the *concept* of *Professional* through these encounters and thus have a broader understanding rather than knowledge that is based on specific cases or situations.

This critical function of concepts, and the fact that a concept can be very meaningful without having a corresponding object, points out some of the difficulties with the views that use a correspondence approach for evaluating the grasp of a concept. The requirement for correspondence was so strict in the writings of Frege and in the early writings of Wittgenstein that concepts that lacked corresponding objects were considered to be without meaning. Concepts such as *Justice*, *Dignity*, *Autonomy*, and many more that are critical not only to nursing but in human existence could not meet this requirement for correspondence.

Research supports some of the challenges with entity views of concepts. Particularly important with regard to concept-based teaching and learning is research in psychology, which raises significant questions about whether the way human beings form concepts is consistent with an entity view (Armstrong, Gleitman, & Gleitman, 1983; Fehr, 1988; McCloskey & Glucksberg, 1978; Medin, 1989; Medin & Schaffer, 1978; Rodgers, 2000). As some of the examples given thus far illustrate, determining the critical characteristics of a concept can be very challenging—so challenging, in fact, that even experts can have difficulty determining what conditions or attributes constitute the clear definition of a concept.

An additional criticism raises concerns in the realm of student assessment. According to an entity view and the idea of specific conditions being necessary to determine that an instance of a particular concept exists, any instance that contains those conditions would count as an example of the concept; no mechanism of judgment or weighting exists that would allow one example to possibly be considered better than another. For teaching and learning purposes, however, and even in everyday life, some situations provide better examples of concepts than others because of the clarity of the presence of the attributes, the significance of the situation, or possibly even the emotional impact and strength of the example overall that leads to a much stronger impression and a greater degree of certainty.

The concept of *Health* provides a good example of this natural variation, along with many other concepts in nursing that are subject to strong individual differences and perceptions. Numerous examples of the concept of *Health* could be presented and, depending on the person being asked, some instances would appear to be better examples than others or would appear to be examples that serve as better prototypes. Nurses are quite familiar with how "health" can be defined very differently by different people based on experience, goals, values, history, and context. Yet examples are sure to exist that are stronger or clearer for many concepts and that provide better examples for teaching purposes, and the faculty would expect a student to recognize such examples. According to an entity view, individual perceptions are not relevant in the definition of a concept and in the identification of instances of a particular concept. Perhaps this characteristic points to one of the most troublesome aspects of an entity view, in that it is not consistent with how people learn and function as members of interactive societies.

In summary, entity views present concepts as objects or things, generally ideas in the mind. A challenge presented by these views is that there is limited explication of how concepts can be examined or evaluated because they are confined to the mind. Linkages between knowledge, learning, language, and behavior are not explicated clearly in discussions of concepts from this perspective. In addition, knowledge is not limited in scope to the physical world, and it changes often; in fact, it must change with new discoveries. As a result, this approach to concepts can be unnecessarily and indefensibly restrictive in many respects.

Dispositional Views of Concepts

Presenting a stark contrast to entity approaches to concepts are what are called dispositional theories of concepts. In a dispositional view, a concept is regarded as a behavior or, more specifically, a capability for a particular behavior rather than as a specific object. One of the behaviors that is important when discussing concepts is the ability to use language effectively. It is essential to have a grasp of a concept in order to communicate.

In a dispositional view, concepts are abstractions, not things themselves. For example, the *concept* of *Bacteria* is not actual bacteria; the concept is a cognitive development based on an understanding of bacteria on an abstract level—in other words, some characteristics that bacteria have in common. Without a firm understanding of the concept, it is not possible to communicate with others about bacteria because each person involved in the conversation could have a radically different understanding of what is meant by the term "bacteria" and the concept that is expressed using that term. It would be essential to discuss a particular bacterium, and not bacteria in general, without a clear concept of *Bacteria*.

According to dispositional views, a solid grasp of a concept enables a person to do more than communicate; the person who understands the concept also is able to perform in certain ways. The nurse who possesses a strong grasp of the concept of *Dignity* will be able to act in ways that preserve or support the dignity of a patient or client, as well as demonstrate his or her own dignity. In another example, a nurse who has a strong grasp of the concept of *Health* will be able to identify things that are examples of health and act in suitable ways (for example, in the promotion of health, assuming that health promotion is a desirable goal). These examples provide a clear picture of some of the strengths of dispositional views, not just in a discipline such as nursing but in everyday life. Health is not a single object; rather, it is something that can be present in varying degrees and in widely different ways in different people and contexts. Health is something that tends to exist more or less. While it may be possible to identify, or at least construct, a single outstanding example of "health," being able to say about a particular instance "this is health" and "this is not health" is not only not realistic but it is not likely to be functional in practical application. There is no single thing that goes by the name "health" that could match a concept of *Health* as needed in an entity view. Even a more tangible and highly familiar object, such as a bird or a dog, can be difficult to delineate conceptually as fully as needed with an entity view. All that is necessary is to consider penguins and the wide variety of canines that exist, from Chihuahuas to mastiffs, and some of the value of seeing concepts as entities that are reflected distinctly in the physical world is muted. Dispositional theories emphasize the behaviors that are possible when someone has a grasp of a concept rather than the ability to identify what is and is not a corresponding object.

The development of dispositional theories was influenced heavily by the writings of Ludwig Wittgenstein in a later phase of his work (Hartnack, 1965). Wittgenstein had been a very strong proponent of correspondence theories earlier in his writings. After being "forced to recognize grave mistakes" (Wittgenstein, 1968, p. vi), he developed a view of concepts based not on rigid criteria but on "family resemblances." As part of this approach, he discussed language games, acknowledging that language is an interactive process: "one party calls out the words, the other acts on them" (Wittgenstein, 1953/1968, p. 5). Language games provide a sort of standard for evaluating speech and language but not a rigid set of criteria as required by correspondence views. Evaluation is based on resemblance—in other words, how well an instance serves as an example of *Health*. This approach provides considerably more flexibility than matching a set of conditions with each situation. A situation can be looked at with some flexibility and variability, thus allowing for concepts to be a little more "fuzzy," without the clear and specific boundaries called for by Essentialism. Although Wittgenstein maintained a focus on language in his later writings, his introduction of the idea of "family resemblances" and language games provided a significant turning point in discussions of concepts toward an emphasis on use rather than matching of necessary and sufficient conditions (Hallett, 1967).

Another philosopher closely associated with dispositional views was Gilbert Ryle (1949, 1971a, 1971b, 1971c, 1971d). Ryle was clear in his description of "use" as a key consideration of concepts: "the use of an expression, or the concept it expresses, is the role it is employed to perform, not any thing or person or event for which it might be supposed to stand" (1971c, p. 364). Ryle's work will be discussed quite superficially here. It is not critical to have an understanding of his catalog of achievements; rather, the point here is to introduce the idea of use and the contributions of this British philosopher to current ideas of concepts. Ryle was very important in overcoming the dualism of earlier philosophers—in other words, the separation of inner and outer realms of existence. Concepts and conceptualization take place in the mind, and there is little disagreement on that point. However, if that is the case, how is it possible to examine or evaluate the concepts that an individual possesses without some means to get inside the mind? Ryle pointed out that thinking, or the process of conceptualization, was manifested in ways that would be examined through mechanisms that were publicly accessible, such as language. Concepts, for Ryle, were not the same as words; words, however, were manifestations of concepts and thus were amenable to examination. If the use of language is considered a form of action or behavior, then it is possible to evaluate conceptual processes, including concept learning, through someone's language, as well as other behaviors.

Essentialism Versus Probabilism

Although the distinctions between dispositional and entity views of concepts are fairly profound, it can be difficult to distinguish the two and place someone who writes about concepts clearly under one heading or the other. Both views hold the same definition of concepts—that they are composed of clusters of attributes. The degree to which those attributes are considered to be rigid with clear boundaries, or not, is a key distinction between the two views. This distinction often has to be determined by identifying the assumptions that underlie a position, such as approaches to concept analysis that are evident in the nursing literature. Another challenge in delineating these two types of views is the fact that concepts vary widely from concrete to more abstract. One end of that continuum is anchored by concepts that have been constructed and stipulated by humans; students are socialized to understand these concepts and associated terminology through their own development processes and formal education. Taxonomies are good examples of these constructed concepts. Because the definitions are stipulated, with very precise criteria, it may be easier to determine whether a specific situation matches the concept. The concept of *Dementia*, for example, might be looked at as if it were an object and can be compared with a situation that is thought to be an example of dementia.

Views of concepts that emphasize correspondence—such that a concept is thought to correspond to some aspect of the real world—have some distinct advantages with regard to teaching and learning and also for application in everyday life. The correspondence view holds that the criteria for determining an instance of a concept are very clear, and thus the ability to determine whether someone possesses a concept of *Dementia* that is "correct" is comparatively simple. The person who possesses the concept of *Dementia* would be able to identify properly what is and is not a case of dementia. For many defined concepts, such as physical phenomena that have clear criteria for their definitions, this advantage seems to be significant. Yet this ability to be clear and specific is a significant limitation of such views, not only for a clinical situation such as one involving a diagnosis but also for physical phenomena that sometimes are less clear than might be expected or acknowledged.

As the example of dementia demonstrates, such clarity can be an illusion. The construction of taxonomies, as a strict form of prescribed definition, often encounters challenges in the attempt to make categories that are mutually exclusive without overlap. In some fields this task is easier to achieve, such as in the classification of biologic organisms (e.g., flowers or insects). In situations involving humans, however—and particularly pronounced in cases of human health—criteria often are presented in the form of a list in which only some of the items on the list must be present for the label to be applicable, thus indicating that there is no single core of characteristics that is captured by the concept. Diagnostic categories change on the basis of new knowledge and changes in social norms, and thus these taxonomies must be reconstructed periodically. Autism is a good example of a situation in which considerable change has occurred over time, resulting in the evolution of the concept to become *Autism Spectrum Disorder*. Taxonomies often function according the idea that it is possible to identify the attributes or characteristics of the concept and that these attributes or characteristics compose a set of "necessary and sufficient conditions," including conditions that must be present (are necessary) and that together are enough (are sufficient) to warrant the taxonomic label. In philosophy this view is known as "essentialism" and is focused on identifying the "essence" of things—in this case, the essence of concepts.

This straightforward desire has much appeal, particularly in areas in which it is essential to label and categorize elements, and it lends a degree of organization that is admirable but not always that easy to achieve. Changes in diagnostic categories, as well as the discovery of new species, reveal the challenges of taxonomy use in a number of different venues. Even some phenomena or entities that seem particularly tangible and clear-cut are subject to change over time such that what was once necessary and sufficient no longer applies. The reclassification of Pluto as a "dwarf planet" rather than a "planet" may be a familiar example (Overbye, 2006).

The essentialist view appears in concept analysis in the search for definitions of concepts such that clear boundaries can be drawn around the concept. In an essentialist approach, it is possible to determine precisely what is and is not an example of the concept of interest. These concepts and their defining attributes also are regarded as universal and unchanging. In one very widely used approach, part of the report of findings of an analysis is to present the concept as it would appear in another context, including contexts that might involve other planets, as one example (Walker & Avant, 1995).

The difficulties with essentialism in regard to concepts are evident in the prior discussion of concepts such as *Dementia* or *Autism*. There may be, for diagnostic purposes, some clear criteria that differentiate when the concept of *Dementia* is and is not appropriately applied. However, in many diagnostic cases, definitions involve a list of numerous attributes, and a subset of those need to be present—for example, three out of six in a list of symptoms. Further, these definitions are constantly changing. Even in cases of diagnostic taxonomies, in which it should be clear whether a condition exists, it is difficult to have the degree of rigidity and universality required of an essentialist view. This approach also assumes that a concept is the same across contexts, including cultural and social contexts, and is not changing, which are two conditions that violate important elements of a nursing perspective. After all, the "essence" of something is what makes it whatever it is. That is, by definition, immutable and unchanging.

In contrast to essentialism, psychologists refer to a "probabilistic" view, reflecting Wittgenstein's idea of family resemblance (Medin, 1989; Smith & Medin, 1981). Other terms for this approach are the "cluster concept" or "prototypical" view. It is also known as "fuzzy set theory" (Armstrong et al., 1983; Fodor & Lepore, 1996; McCloskey & Glucksberg, 1978). As the terminology indicates, these approaches to concepts recognize that boundaries are not always clear, that context can make a difference in interpretation, and that some instances of concepts serve as better examples (prototypes) than others. Some concepts are amenable, at least on a short-term basis (barring future change), to clearer boundaries and more consistency across examples. Nurses study and work with human beings, however, and even some of the more "scientific" aspects, such as the nature of disease and what constitutes "cure," along with many of the relevant concepts, are subject to considerable variation and change over time. Even if a definition can be based on necessary and sufficient conditions for a period, such as the concept of *Anaphylactic Shock*, the potential still exists for the conceptual definition to change as knowledge grows with respect to the phenomenon. Some concepts will change more often or more quickly than others, but the probability of conceptual change must be kept in mind when developing curricula for a conceptual approach to teaching.

What Does This Mean for Concept-Based Teaching?

Effective teaching in a concept-based curriculum requires an understanding of the different perspectives that exist about concepts. The assumptions that are made about the nature of concepts and their role in the discipline undoubtedly affect the teaching strategies that are used in a concept-based approach to nursing education. The previous discussion reveals some of the array of approaches that exist in philosophy and how those approaches may affect or be manifested in nursing education.

Clarity Regarding Terminology

At the most basic level, clarity about terminology is important. Faculty who teach any curriculum need to be clear in how they use words to describe certain phenomena. This clarity is particularly critical when talking about areas that are replete with ambiguity and confusion, as is the case with theoretical ideas such as concepts. The definition given previously, that concepts are clusters of attributes that are abstracted from phenomena and given an associated term for expression, is simple, complete, and broadly applicable to concepts of all types (Rodgers, 2000).

It is important to further differentiate some aspects of concepts that can be confusing. First, the concept is the idea, not the actual object. Instruments, tools, and physical implements used in nursing are mechanisms to measure abstract concepts. A thermometer is a tool to measure *Temperature*, and *Temperature* is a concept. In teaching, it is important to be distinct about the abstract idea (concept) and the physical embodiment of that concept. *Thermometer* also can be a concept—that is, the concept of *Thermometer*—if discussion is about thermometers in regard to the characteristics that make something a thermometer. As noted previously in the discussion of dogs, there are dogs, and there is the *concept* of *Dogs*, which need to be acknowledged as being different things. Teaching about the physical entities known as dogs will be very different from teaching that addresses dogs on a conceptual level. Awareness of that distinction is critical to effective concept-based teaching.

Concepts and Constructs

Concepts also can be clustered to form constructs. When teaching and developing curricula, it is important to recognize the base elements—that is, the most simple concepts—along with what are more properly regarded as constructs. Concept-based teaching may be focused on both. For example, *Thermoregulation* includes the concepts of *Regulation,* as well as concepts related to *Temperature, Heat, Cold,* and *Measurement.* In the majority of cases, constructs can be addressed in teaching in the same manner as concepts. However, it may be helpful to address the basic elements of such constructs to assist students in learning.

Concepts and Context

Concepts also are combined, sometimes, into theory. A common misconception in nursing is based on the often-repeated statement that "concepts are the building blocks of theory" (Rodgers & Knafl, 2000). Although this statement is true, theories are constructed through the identification of relationships among concepts, and this ubiquitous statement gives the impression that concepts are not of value unless they are in the context of theory. The theoretical literature in nursing is focused on the weaving together of concepts to make theory. What is lost in this process is the recognition that concepts themselves are theoretical products. As is evident in the discussion of philosophy earlier in this chapter, concepts are very powerful theoretical elements that carry with them the influences of society, history, culture, disciplines, and existing knowledge. In other words, concepts are contextually bound. Attempts to view them as universal or as the same regardless of context will undermine a primary value of nursing with regard to the uniqueness of each individual. There is such a thing as the concept of *Health*. What will be considered to be the attributes of the concept of *Health,* and thus suitable examples of the concept, will vary widely across contexts.

The Need for a Consistent Philosophical Approach

Consistency in the philosophical approach to concepts that underlie a concept-based curriculum can be very helpful to students as they proceed with their conceptual learning. It is tempting at times to see some concepts as static, with clear boundaries, and with obvious and clear examples of appropriate use. In such a situation, teaching and assessment of learning should be consistent with that approach. Yet it is obvious in some of the previous examples that this approach does not fit all concepts. Shifting philosophical perspectives—that is, seeing some concepts as rigid and static and others as always changing and "fuzzy"—would call for very different teaching and evaluation strategies. Ultimately, this approach could be very confusing to students and gives the impression that faculty are a bit confused about what concepts are and how learning should be evaluated.

Such an approach is contradictory because it requires the use of two ideas about concepts that are very much in conflict. A concept cannot be both static and rigid *and* fuzzy and dynamic. A concept cannot be composed of necessary and sufficient conditions yet also not be so constructed. When looking at individual concepts, the possibility of considerable certainty may seem to exist. For example, it should be easy enough to determine when sepsis exists and when it is not present. Yet even the most concrete of concepts will have some variation either across humans or over time. The possibility and the likelihood of change over time must be acknowledged for all concepts.

Rather than adopt competing viewpoints about concepts—a rigid one for those that are more clear and a fuzzy view for those that are more abstract or less refined—with the confusion that undoubtedly would result in the minds of the students (and probably faculty as well), another option may be utilized. Concepts can be viewed with use of a consistent and defensible philosophy that acknowledges that they occupy a continuum of characteristics: concrete to abstract, well developed to amorphous, widely fluctuating over time and context to relatively stable. Philosophical consistency is important in having a cogent and coherent approach to the curriculum. Students will benefit from a clear understanding of what a concept is, what constitutes the definition, and how concepts can be evaluated, while acknowledging that some will be more concrete and better developed than others. Morse (1995) discussed this in regard to how "mature" the concept is. However, it has nothing to do with maturity or longevity; it has to do with the strength of evidence and the comfort level with which certain concepts are embraced in nursing. Some aspects of existence are less subject to fluctuation and change than are others. For example, it is quite clear what hypertension is, yet there will always be people who, no matter how clear the definition might be, present variations of this otherwise very clear condition. Labile hypertension has been considered a separate class, yet evidence indicates that all hypertension shows some lability. Some disease conditions that seem very obvious end up having different origins—for example, the discovery of *Helicobacter pylori* as a causative agent for peptic ulcers. It was "known" with great certainty what caused such ulcers…until the evidence became overwhelming that the widely accepted certainty was not so certain after all.

So, for persons teaching according to concept-based curricula, it is important to be consistent with the view of concepts that underlies the curriculum and with how each instructor or faculty member presents that view in different learning encounters. A defensible view of concepts must allow for processes of conceptual change. In fact, promoting awareness of processes of conceptual change in students can help strengthen a value for keeping up with current literature and discoveries. A shortcoming of education regardless of the approach can be the imparted belief that there is such a thing as proof or "Truth;" in the case of concept-based curricula, ample opportunities exist to reinforce the common nature of conceptual change.

Assessment must be consistent with the philosophical view of concepts and the nature of the particular conceptual learning that is being evaluated. Teaching conceptually but testing specific details or "facts" will send a contradictory message to students regarding the importance of conceptual understanding in nursing. It also is likely to skew assessment results because the mode of teaching will not be consistent with the form of evaluation or measurement. Consequently, a critical issue in effective concept-based teaching is the determination of how understanding can be evaluated appropriately, which can vary with the origin, nature, specificity, clarity, and subjective nature of specific concepts.

Concepts Grounded in Nursing Discipline

Finally, it is important to recognize that concept-based teaching must be grounded in the specific conceptual base of the discipline of nursing. In selecting the concepts to be included in the curriculum, and in discriminating among closely related concepts, students are being socialized into the discipline and profession of nursing. Toulmin (1972) argued that a distinguishing feature of a discipline, and an important element in its continuity over generations, is the "conceptual repertoire" that forms a "transmit" in regard to both knowledge and socialization. Recognizing that concept-based teaching has a particularly strong role in development of the student as a professional nurse places a strong burden on the curriculum and faculty but is also an outstanding opportunity for shaping the future of the discipline.

Summary

A concept-based approach to teaching in nursing offers a number of advantages as an educational model for student learning. For such an approach to be successful, however, it is essential that the faculty have an understanding of the nature of concepts and how they function in the process of learning and be consistent in the selection and implementation of a philosophical viewpoint about concepts. Faculty also need to recognize the importance of conceptual change in the discipline and connect that to evidence-based practice. Doing so will provide the students not only with a foundation of concepts essential for nursing practice but an appreciation for adapting to new developments in the discipline as they arise. Concepts lose their value if they are seen as static entities to be memorized and matched up with segments of reality. Grasping and applying concepts, and using the appropriate language to express them, is a dynamic process that empowers the students not only to perform at high levels but to keep current with new developments as they pursue their careers in nursing.

REFERENCES

Aristotle: Posterior Analytics. (G. R. G. Mure, Trans.). In McKeon R, editor: *Introduction to Aristotle*, New York, NY, 1947, Random House, pp 9–109.

Aristotle: Categories. (J. L. Ackrill, Trans.). In Barnes J, editor: *The complete works of Aristotle*, Princeton, NJ, 1984, Princeton University, pp 3–24.

Armstrong SL, Gleitman LR, Gleitman H: What some concepts might not be, *Cognition* 13:263–308, 1983.

Chinn PL, Kramer MK: *Theory and nursing: A systematic approach*, 3rd ed., St. Louis, MO, 1991, Mosby.

Chinn PL, Kramer MK: *Integrated theory and knowledge development in nursing*, 8th ed., St. Louis, MO, 2011, Elsevier.

Cowles KV, Rodgers BL: The concept of grief: An evolutionary perspective. In Rodgers BL, Knafl KA, editors: *Concept development in nursing: Foundations, techniques, and applications*, 2nd ed., Philadelphia, PA, 2000, WB Saunders, pp 103–117.

Descartes R: Meditations on first philosophy. In Beardsley MC, editor: *The European philosophers from Descartes to Nietzsche*, New York, NY, 1960, Random House, pp 25–96 (Original work published 1644).

Diers D: *Research in nursing practice*, Philadelphia, PA, 1979, J. B. Lippincott.

Fehr B: Prototype analysis of the concepts of love and commitment, *Journal of Personality and Social Psychology* 55:557–579, 1988.

Fodor J, Lepore E: The red herring and the pet fish: Why concepts still can't be prototypes, *Cognition* 58:253–270, 1996.

Frege G: Grundgesetze der Arithmetic. (P. T. Geach, Trans.). In Geach P, Black M, editors: *Translations from the philosophical writings of Gottlob Frege*, Oxford, 1952a, Basil Blackwell, pp 159–181.

Frege G: On concept and object. (P. T. Geach, Trans.). In Geach P, Black M, editors: *Translations from the philosophical writings of Gottlob Frege*, Oxford, 1952b, Basil Blackwell, pp 42–55.

Hallett G: *Wittgenstein's definition of meaning as use*, New York, NY, 1967, Fordham University.

Hardy MK: Theories: Components, development, evaluation, *Nursing Research* 23:100–107, 1974.

Hartnack J: *Wittgenstein and modern philosophy* (M. Cranston, Trans.). New York, NY, 1965, New York University.

Kant I: *Critique of pure reason* (N. K. Smith, Trans.). New York, NY, 1965, St. Martin's Press (Original work published 1781).

King IM: Concepts: Essential elements of theories, *Nursing Science Quarterly* 1:22–25, 1988.

Lizardo O: Re-conceptualizing abstract conceptualization in social theory: The case of the "structure" concept, *Journal for the Theory of Social Behavior* 43(2):155–180, 2013.

Locke J: *An essay concerning human understanding*, Oxford, 1975, Oxford University (Original work published 1690).

Mahon BZ, Caramazza A: Concepts and categories: A cognitive neuropsychological perspective, *Annual Review of Psychology* 60:27–51, 2009.

McCloskey ME, Glucksberg S: Natural categories: Well defined or fuzzy sets? *Memory & Cognition* 6:462–472, 1978.

Medin DL: Concepts and conceptual structure, *American Psychologist* 44:1469–1481, 1989.

Medin DL, Schaffer MM: Context theory of classification learning, *Psychological Review* 85:207–238, 1978.

Meleis AI: *Theoretical nursing*, 2nd ed., Philadelphia, PA, 1991, J. B. Lippincott.

Meleis AI: *Theoretical nursing*, 3rd ed., Philadelphia, PA, 1997, J. B. Lippincott.

Meleis AI: *Theoretical nursing*, 5th ed., Philadelphia, PA, 2012, Lippincott Williams & Wilkins.

Morse MM: Exploring the theoretical basis of nursing knowledge using advanced techniques of concept analysis, *Advances in Nursing Science* 17(3):31–46, 1995.

Norris CM: *Concept clarification in nursing*, Rockville, MD, 1982, Aspen.

Overbye D: *Pluto is demoted to "dwarf planet."*, New York Times, 2006 August 24. Available online http://www.nytimes.com/2006/08/24/science/space/25pluto.html?_r=0Rodgers, B. L. (1989). Concepts, analysis, and the development of nursing knowledge: The evolutionary cycle. *Journal of Advanced Nursing*, 14, 330–335.

Rodgers BL: Philosophical foundations of concept development. In Rodgers BL, Knafl KA, editors: *Concept Development in Nursing: Foundations, techniques, and applications*, Philadelphia, PA, 2000, W. B. Saunders, pp 7–37.

Rodgers BL, Knafl KA: Introduction to concept development in nursing. In Rodgers BL, Knafl KA, editors: *Concept Development in Nursing: Foundations, techniques, and applications*, Philadelphia, PA, 2000, W. B. Saunders, pp 1–6.

Ryle G: *The concept of mind*, Chicago, IL, 1949, University of Chicago.

Ryle G: Systematically misleading expressions, *Collected papers*, Vol. 2. London, 1971a, Hutchinson. 39–62.

Ryle G: The theory of meaning, *Collected papers*, Vol. 2. London, 1971b, Hutchinson. 350–372.

Ryle G: Thinking thoughts and having concepts, *Collected papers*, Vol. 2. London, 1971c, Hutchinson. 446–450.

Ryle G: Use, usage and meaning, *Collected papers*, Vol. 2. London, 1971d, Hutchinson. 407–414.

Smith EE, Medin DL: *Categories and concepts*, Cambridge, MA, 1981, Harvard University.

Sundbo DIC: Local food: The social construction of a concept, Section B., Soil and plant science *Acta Agriculturae Scandinavica* 63(Supp1):66–77, 2013.

Toulmin S: *Human understanding*, Princeton, NJ, 1972, Princeton University.

Walker LO, Avant KC: *Strategies for theory construction in nursing*, 2nd ed., Norwalk, CT, 1988, Appleton & Lange.

Walker LO, Avant KC: *Strategies for theory construction in nursing*, 3rd ed., Norwalk, CT, 1995, Appleton & Lange.

Walker LO, Avant KC: *Strategies for theory construction in nursing*, 5th ed., Boston, MA, 2011, Prentice-Hall.

Watson J: *Nursing: The philosophy and science of caring*, Boston, MA, 1979, Little, Brown.

Wittgenstein L: *Philosophical investigations*, G. E. M. Anscombe, Trans), 3rd ed., New York, NY, 1968, Macmillan (Original work published 1953).

Development of Concepts for Concept-Based Teaching

3

Beth Rodgers

A general overview of ideas associated with concepts as a foundation for understanding the nature and use of concepts was presented in Chapter 2. Exploration of the philosophical foundation of concepts was a particular focus because understanding the variety of approaches to concepts has a clear impact on concept-based teaching. It is important that instructors working with concept-based curricula understand the confusion that exists regarding what a concept is, as well as the many different approaches to concepts. The perspective taken by the faculty, and represented by the curriculum overall, can have a profound effect on student learning and on how concept-based teaching occurs.

Based on the philosophical perspective that underlies the curriculum and the shared vision of concepts, faculty need to determine not only which concepts are relevant to the curriculum but what should be the focus of each aspect of the curriculum in terms of definitions, use, and language, for example. Once those decisions are made, there will be a shared foundation for moving forward with the construction of appropriate learning activities. At that point, faculty members are confronted with a challenging and multifaceted task. For each chosen concept in the curriculum, a number of aspects need to be considered: What is a "conceptually adequate definition"? In what settings do instances of the concept occur? What effect does context/setting/user have on the concept? What other concepts are similar, related, or easily confused with the concept of interest? How is that concept expressed or shared or discussed with others? What means are appropriate to assess a student's "grasp" of the concept? Other chapters in this text deal with various aspects of these challenges. In this chapter, the focus is on definitions, relationships among concepts, and language, as these components are critical to the formation of learning and assessment strategies as a foundation for developing and implementing a sound curriculum for concept-based teaching.

Conceptually Adequate Definitions

The idea of "definition" is a familiar one to all language holders. In regard to words (rather than referring to the distinctness or sharpness of the edges of an object or illustration), definitions can be found quite readily in any dictionary. The definition of "definition" is "a statement of the exact meaning of a word, especially in a dictionary…. An exact statement or description of the nature, scope, or meaning of something." (*Oxford Dictionary of English*, 2005, p. 455). In simple terms, a definition of a word is the "meaning" of that word, similar to its reference or proper use in a sentence. Philosophers have discussed for centuries the idea of "meaning," but this common idea of definition and meaning is much more simple. Knowing the definition of a word enables the language holder to use that word effectively in a sentence and, if the person on the receiving end understands that definition, that individual can understand the original speaker or writer. When one considers the number of homonyms in the English language, the need for definitions becomes even clearer (Box 3-1). Homonyms also point out the importance of making a distinction between concepts and the words that are used to express those concepts. The words may be the same, but in many cases, the concepts expressed by the word can be very different.

Definitions typically are written as declarative statements and often as sentence fragments, such as the definition of "grief" presented in the *Oxford Dictionary of English* (2005): "intense sorrow, especially caused by someone's death." It also is defined in this same source as "an instance or cause of intense sorrow" (p. 762). Such definitions, when shared, make communication possible on a general level. But they also present a lot of questions that indicate how that communication may not be as common as desired. In regard to developing a knowledge base, or using

---

BOX 3-1 **Homonyms**

A homonym is a word with the same spelling and pronunciation but with different definitions. A homonym does not usually express the same *concept*. Each use of the term must be associated with a different concept and conceptual definition for correct application. Consider all the following applications for the concept of *Bill*:

- Money; a dollar bill
- The part of a bird's jaw with a horny covering; a beak
- An itemized statement of fees or charges
- The visor portion of a cap
- A common first name
- A draft of proposed law presented for legislation

an idea or phenomenon definitively in research or theory, the problems should be obvious. What counts as "intense sorrow"? According to this dictionary, grief is "especially caused by someone's death." Are there other causes? Can intense sorrow stem from some other type of loss? What are the differences between sorrow and anguish, despair, and hopelessness? Do people act out their grief in different ways, and is it still "grief" if the behaviors differ? Such questions reveal how unclear our terminology really is sometimes and the challenges that terminology can present in nursing situations.

Conceptual definitions work in a similar manner but require a greater degree of specificity. As pointed out in Chapter 2, a concept is composed of a set of attributes. A conceptual definition, therefore, is the clear statement of those attributes. The impact of the philosophy underlying this idea of definition should be obvious, yet it is worth focusing on for a bit more discussion. A definition can be considered "conceptually adequate" when it stipulates the components of the concept with sufficient clarity that the concept can be used effectively (Rodgers, 2000). A philosophical approach to concepts that is based on ideas about correspondence will require a definition that includes the attributes that are essential to identify the aspect of the real world that corresponds to the concept. For example, the concept of *Sepsis* in such a view must be defined by stipulating the attributes that are essential to identify, without a doubt, an instance of actual sepsis. This definition is composed of the conditions that are necessary and sufficient to identify an instance of the concept and that hold across a variety of contexts. A definition that falls short of this goal might still be of some use; for example, it might give some idea about what reasonably can be conceptualized as *Sepsis*, but it would leave multiple aspects of the concept open to debate. Therefore, it would not be an adequate definition or, more specifically, a "conceptually adequate" definition.

Conceptual Change Over Time

As noted previously, the idea that concepts can be defined by necessary and sufficient conditions, at first glance, does seem to fit some of the ideas that are critical to nursing knowledge (Walker & Avant, 2011). But there are numerous instances where this is not consistent. Further, even for those instances that do seem to fit at present, the possibility and in fact the likelihood of change in the future needs to be instilled in students as a reminder to keep up to date with the latest knowledge. History is full of examples of situations in which there seemed good reason to believe that certainty had been achieved only to have that certainty questioned over time. A more contemporary view of concepts allows for this evolution and focuses on the use of concepts rather than on correspondence theory (Rodgers, 2000). This view is not only philosophically sound but also a good fit with concept-based teaching. A student could be very adept at reciting facts and listing details and principles, but if the student cannot apply that knowledge in real-life situations, the learning is of no value. It is the use of concepts that makes it clear whether the student has a full grasp of the essential knowledge. It is not sufficient in nursing to merely "know" something; rather, it is essential that the nurse be able to apply that knowledge, recognize subtle nuances and variations in application across multiple settings and situations, evaluate the application, and alter that knowledge based on evaluation and as new quality information becomes available. The approach to concepts and concept-based teaching that is used in nursing education must be one that promotes the attainment of those goals.

The Need for Conceptual Clarity

A critical aspect in this process is determining how concepts will be presented in the curriculum—in other words, what will constitute a "conceptually adequate" approach for the purposes of the educational setting. Identifying concepts that are essential to the discipline and then providing students with a list of essential attributes, thus invoking the idea of "necessary and sufficient conditions" described in the previous chapter, is not consistent with the ideology just described. This approach gives students the impression that concepts are static and perfectly clear, with distinguishable boundaries, and with consistency regardless of context or situation. This approach promotes memorization rather than application, because students undoubtedly will be focused on learning the essential attributes so those can be recited at a later time (for example, on multiple choice tests). This approach also fails to acknowledge the critical and essential processes of application and also of conceptual change.

What is needed for teaching purposes (and for concept development in general) is a way to identify and communicate the core features of a concept while allowing for important considerations such as application, variation across contexts, conceptual change, and the fact that concepts are never perfect or fully finished products, nor are they always perfectly distinct from each other. These observations must not be seen as shortcomings; rather, they are critical aspects of concepts that enable the growth and change that is essential to dynamic application and that allow for variations across cultures, contexts, and individuals. It is the more rigid approach that actually possesses far greater shortcomings, even though the illusion of clarity and exactness may be comforting to student and instructor alike. It might be highly desirable to "know," ultimately and without question, what really constitutes the concepts of *Dignity* or *Peptic Ulcer*. Yet both of these concepts must be amenable to variation across individuals, cultures, contexts, and the variation required by new discoveries. As with all concepts, both *Dignity* and *Peptic Ulcer* have needed to change as society has changed and as new research forced reconsideration and further development of these concepts.

Before moving on to a discussion of the "how to" of arriving at useful conceptually adequate definitions, it is worth pointing out the confusion that often results when discussing definition and meaning. Definitions, regardless of context, are inherently different from meaning, and caution should be exercised so the two ideas are not confused. A "conceptually adequate definition" was explained previously but will be reiterated here for the sake of clarity. It is the illumination of the key components of a concept such that its core attributes and contextual aspects are evident and sufficient to differentiate the concept from those that may exist with some relationship to the concept of interest. In colloquial terms, and when learning vocabulary, it is common to ask what a particular word "means," and yet meaning and definition are very different ideas (different concepts). Although occasionally a philosopher will use the terms "meaning" and "definition" as if they are similar, a wide array of thought exists that addresses "meaning" in regard to a subjective, personal, experiential interpretation of an event or phenomenon. For example, the concept of *Pain* can be defined in a particular way with regard to its attributes, context, and use. The meaning of that pain will vary across individuals with regard to whether the individual sees pain as transformative, a learning experience, punishment, something to be avoided at all costs, something that provides an opportunity for increased spiritual awareness, and other possible individual interpretations. Keeping in mind the distinction between definition and meaning, and using those ideas judiciously, can help students not only learn the concepts by virtue of their definitions but also gain a range of application by understanding the potential for variations in meaning across different individuals and contexts.

Procedures for Concept Analysis and Clarification

The process of identifying the core components of a concept is concept clarification, which most commonly is accomplished by using methods of concept analysis. Concept analysis should be viewed as a useful step in a larger process of concept development. Various forms of inquiry, such as traditional scientific work, all contribute to knowledge related to the concepts being studied. Research of many types helps to clarify and expand knowledge about the subject being studied. On one level, this is all part of the process of concept development, not merely the generation of new information or "facts." Theory development also requires attention to concepts, and often the process of concept development is a major focus of expanding and clarifying an existing theory. Keeping concept analysis within the broader context of concept development will help students remember that concepts are not static and that they, too, can continue to develop their own

---

BOX 3-2 **Approaches to Concept Analysis Used in Nursing**

- Morse (1995) – Principle-Based Concept Analysis
- Norris (1982) — Concept Clarification
- Walker and Avant (1983, 2011) – Concept Analysis
- Rodgers (1989, 2000) – Evolutionary Cycle of Concept Development
- Schwartz-Barcott and Kim (1986) – Hybrid Model of Concept Development

---

concepts as they apply and evaluate their own conceptual knowledge. The analysis of concepts is a beneficial and often a critical starting point in this process.

Concept analysis is well established in the literature of nursing, and several different methodologies exist for this purpose. Box 3-2 contains a list of some of the methodologies that have been used in nursing studies. Until recently, however, little information was available that would help researchers or others interested in this type of work identify and design a methodologically and philosophically sound approach. It is not uncommon in the literature to find that authors followed a particular approach because it was recommended by an instructor, it was found frequently in the literature, or it seemed easy to follow (Rodgers, 2000). Convenience and commonality, however, are not appropriate criteria for selecting a procedure for inquiry. Exploring concepts for purposes of concept-based teaching may not be formal research, but it still calls for rigorous and sound inquiry. Similarly, the process and the presentation of the concept need to be consistent with the philosophical approach to concepts that is represented throughout the curriculum.

In selecting the approach to clarify a concept for purposes of concept-based teaching, the instructor also should consider the nature of the concept to be analyzed. As described elsewhere, some concepts are capable of more specificity, such as those that are represented by diagnostic criteria or taxonomies. The detail and specificity may be easier to achieve with concepts that are newer as they typically do not evidence a long history of conceptual change. It also may be possible to identify physical or tangible objects that serve as examples of such concepts, which can make clarification and description easier to accomplish, keeping in mind actual objects that represent the concept. An example of such a concept would be *Bacteria,* which has a specific, clear, and easily discernible definition. Physiologic concepts, in general, will be amenable to more precision, whereas concepts pertaining to intangible qualities such as emotion, behavior, and social phenomena (the psychosocial concepts) are going to show more variation and vagueness. Morse, Mitcham, Hupcey, and Tason (1996) referred to some concepts as being "mature" in reference to the length of their existence and presumed state of development. It is often assumed that more mature concepts are capable of greater precision because of their longevity. However, a lengthy period of use only exposes a concept to more change and variation, and sometimes to radical change. While the history of the emergence and evolution of a concept can shed a great deal of light on its definition and use over time, it is not an essential consideration in deciding how to proceed with concept development.

Evolutionary Model of Concept Development

For the purposes of concept-based teaching, especially instilling in students an appreciation for conceptual change over time, the approach to concept clarification based on the Evolutionary Model of Concept Development (Rodgers, 2000) is very useful and consistent with contemporary philosophical views of concepts. In this model, clarification of a concept serves as an important step in a broader process of concept development. It is desirable that students not only understand important concepts but that they see their application of concepts as feeding back into the developmental process. Analysis is the starting point in an ongoing cycle of concept development.

Processes of concept analysis, regardless of philosophical orientation, have many common features. A concept is, by definition, composed of a cluster of attributes; analysis is, by definition, the process of breaking something down to identify its constituent components (Rodgers, 2000). Therefore, concept analysis is the process of breaking a concept down to identify the attributes that constitute its definition. In this model, concepts are considered to have a particular "use"—that is, the common construction of the concept, the terminology that is associated with it, and the contexts to which it typically is applied. The process of analysis can be focused on this use, with instances of use examined to identify the attributes and other characteristics of the concept that aid in clarification. For the purposes of concept-based teaching, the most likely sources of data for examining the use of the concept will be the professional literature, such as publications in nursing and related journals. Concepts also are expressed in other forms, such as through spoken language and even through the performing arts. For teaching purposes, however, the appropriate starting point is the professional literature. For some concepts, it also can be illuminating to examine popular constructions of a concept, particularly for those that can have a strong individual interpretation or cultural and contextual variation. The concept of *Grief*, for example, not only has a large base of professional literature but can be found in a wide array of popular literature as well. Understanding these perspectives, as expressed by people experiencing the concept, can provide important insights to help the student apply the concept and understand variations in the concept across settings and situations.

Using the Evolutionary Model for Teaching

The Evolutionary Model is associated with a formal process of concept analysis that can be used in a thorough attempt at concept clarification for the purposes of teaching. This approach looks similar to the one advocated by the popular writings of Walker and Avant (2011). In fact, all approaches to concept analysis have a great deal in common with regard to the specific activities that are conducted as part of the analysis. There are, however, what may seem subtle but actually are quite profound differences. A detailed discussion of the differences is beyond the scope of this chapter but can be found in Rodgers (2000).

The Evolutionary Model is not a variant of approaches based on the work of Wilson (1963), such as that proposed by Walker and Avant. For purposes of developing clear concepts for concept-based teaching, the process identified in the following sections can be very effective. Note that it also can be used in teaching, taking students through the process of the analysis to ensure that all of the components of the concept are presented clearly through the learning experience. For a thorough discussion of this approach, please see the description provided elsewhere (Rodgers, 2000). A simplified version, intended for ease of use by instructors and faculty, is provided here.

 Misconceptions and Clarifications

Misconception: The various approaches to concept analysis found in the literature are essentially the same.	**Clarification:** The various approaches to concept analysis appear similar in many ways, but the differences actually are quite profound.

Identifying the Concept of Interest

First, it is essential to identify the concept of interest. The emphasis needs to be on the idea that is communicated, not the word that is used to discuss it. Words are expressions of ideas, not the ideas themselves. Using the example of *Grief* again, the instructor needs to determine what term best expresses the concept to be discussed. Some obvious possibilities include *Bereavement* and *Loss*. *Grief* also might be discussed in the context of stress, coping, adaptation, resilience, and other terms that express related ideas. It is important to be clear about what the concept of interest is and then what term is best used to express that concept. The selection of the term will guide the clarification process, along with any teaching and learning interactions with students. As the example of grief indicates, there may be two terms that seem to express similar ideas, and it may be appropriate to explore both to determine which term is most appropriate and has the broadest support. The terms "grief" and "bereavement" both have relevance in the exploration of the same concept, although a thorough review of the literature does reveal some differences (Rodgers & Cowles, 2000).

Another example of a situation in which the selection of the concept and associated terminology is critical to conceptual understanding is the concept of adherence, also referred to as "compliance" (Bissonnette, 2013). Conceptually, the difference is relatively minor, with the term "adherence" substituted for "compliance" in an effort to diminish what seemed like the "more paternalistic" (pp. 53-54) approach associated with "compliance." It is debatable whether the concept itself actually changed with this alteration in terminology. It would be an important aspect to explore, acknowledging the controversy and contrasts, when working with students who are learning this concept. This serves as a good example of how the selection of terminology is important in identifying examples of the concept as a literature search for "compliance" may not reveal the very closely related literature of "adherence." This example also points out that the concept and not the term must be the focus of attention, or a considerable amount of important information could be excluded from the learning experience. Discussion of the concept, along with both terms, is important to promoting the students' grasp of the concept and their ability to use it effectively.

Determine the Relevant Context

Second, the process of concept clarification and development requires attention to the context of the use of the concept. The concept of compliance or adherence, however it is expressed, may be different in health care than it is in an engineering application—or it may not be different. A more obvious example is the concept of coping. In a health care context, coping refers to behavioral and cognitive means of adjusting to various situations. *Coping,* as a concept, involves not only a positive outcome, as in, "She is coping well with her new challenges," but the process of making responses to changing stimuli. *Coping* often is discussed in health care in the context of concepts such as *Stress, Adaptation,* and *Resilience* (Buchanan, 2013). The term "coping" also can be found in regard to woodworking, such as "coping saw" (Walker & Avant, 2011). In some respects, this concept is similar, because the saw makes precise and fine adjustments to produce intricate patterns in the material being cut. The saw makes it possible for wood, for example, to respond to its surroundings to make a precise fit. Walker and Avant (2011) also identify "coping" in reference to a type of garment and refer to all of these examples as varied uses of the same concept, arguing that all of the examples should be included in the analysis. This approach would be misleading on a number of levels, however, because these uses and ideas of coping clearly miss the intricacies and important aspects of coping as a psychological and cognitive process (Giddens & Edds, 2013; Rodgers, 2000). Further, this approach is a solid example of confusing terminology, or the use of a word, with the use of a concept. Keeping the focus on the concept of *Coping*, which, for nursing purposes, is used and discussed in regard to a distinct type of human experience, will help students focus and ensure a clear emphasis on the concept of interest rather than on the terminology. Settings and application also may include considerations about age, culture, and care context, to the extent that those considerations are relevant. These applications are just a few in a long list of possible applications that exist for many concepts of interest in nursing.

It is important at this stage to point out that even though the activities are enumerated here, thus giving the impression that they occur in sequential fashion, the process of concept clarification is not a linear process at all. Each activity discussed can be affected by all of the others; for example, determining what terminology will work best for a literature review will be affected by the literature that is uncovered during the review. This terminology may again need to be changed as literature is reviewed. It is important to see the flow of activities as an iterative process, with each activity influenced by the others.

Collect Data to Clarify the Concept

Data collection proceeds once some of the critical decisions about the concept have been made, at least on a preliminary basis. As previously noted, data collection may lead the faculty to look at other terminology, sources, or contexts. Consequently, even though data collection is a major focus of the analysis and development processes, it is not an isolated endeavor that is pursued without regard for the other parts of the process. For concept-based teaching, data collection will be focused on collecting sufficient information to determine the major components of the concept. These components include the attributes of the concept—in other words, its key components—along with discussion of the context in which the concept is used. Context can include social and cultural considerations in addition to elements that reflect a time sequence. Situations or events that occur before an instance of the concept and those that occur after are typically discussed as "antecedents" and "consequences," respectively. For purposes of concept-based teaching, these situations or events might be more appropriately discussed in a general time sequence as precursors or "causes," if appropriate, or other terminology consistent with a clinical application, and consequences can be discussed as outcomes or sequelae or simply as consequences. Antecedents and consequences help to put the concept in an application setting so that students can understand not just the concept but when they might see examples of it and what creates a situation in which the concept is applicable, along with possible outcomes. Data that help answer these questions are derived from the literature and then are analyzed to develop clear indicators of the effective use of the concept. Proceeding in this manner reveals the "state of the science" regarding the concept for nursing application (Rodgers, 2000).

Identify Exemplars

Finally, exemplars of the proper use of the concept help students grasp the application of the concept in the appropriate context and make the concept "come to life." Exemplars, in this view, are not the same as "model cases." A model case, according to Wilson (1963), is a case "which we are absolutely sure" is an instance of the concept in that it contains all of the conditions that are "necessary and sufficient" to comprise an example of the concept (p. 28). Walker and Avant (2011) include these, and other types of cases, in their approach to analysis. There is a significant problem with "model" cases, however, in that they may give the impression of greater clarity and certainty than is appropriate. The term "exemplar" is used purposefully in the Evolutionary Method to reflect the fact that these examples ideally can be found in "real life" and are not models or paradigmatic cases that are constructed by the person doing the analysis (Fehr, 1988; Rodgers, 2000). Multiple examples can be used to show the nuances of the concept in different applications and contexts and to help students accept how boundaries more often are fuzzy and unclear than distinct and rigid. Exemplars that show changes over time and the influence of new research can be an important part of nursing socialization and help students gain an appreciation for evidence-based practice and how the evidence often is changing. Concepts related to sleep, for example, have changed considerably in recent years as sleep has become an established specialty area and as knowledge has changed about the importance of sleep and various disruptors. The concept of *Sleep* can be discussed in the context of differentiation from fatigue, as a factor in metabolic regularity, in relation to sleep-disordered breathing, and in association with cognitive functioning, to name just a few examples of how sleep is of concern. As another example, the concept of *Infection* is one that nurses work with frequently, and it may be discussed with regard to a patient who has an infectious process and with regard to primary prevention. As part of this process, it may be beneficial to point out where there is a need for further knowledge development or research and where vague areas and questions remain regarding the concept. The more that students can be helped to see how knowledge constantly changes and to view all sides of a concept and a wide array of applications, the more they are likely to be able to think critically and creatively and solve problems in actual clinical application.

Bringing the Concept Presentation to Life

The results of concept analysis, when reported in the literature, may seem very tedious or cumbersome to read. There typically is a listing of each of the major components with varying amounts of discussion about each component. For purposes of inquiry, where it is necessary to be clear about the status of each component of the concept to identify directions for future development, this information may be useful. For education, however, it is more important that the concept be presented in a way that comes alive for students. The necessary degree of conceptual clarity must be present, but the analysis and presentation will be more effective if the components are woven together in a manner that helps students grasp the appearance and use of the concept in real-life situations.

The intent of concept clarification activities in a concept-based curriculum is to help the students grasp the concept and be able to use it effectively. This includes giving students sufficient information to (1) recognize the occurrence of the concept and be clear and appropriate in its application; (2) value the contextual elements; (3) recognize and use associated terminology; (4) explore distinctions among similar concepts; and (5) appreciate the nuances and subtleties of the concept and its areas of imperfection. There is no limit to how a concept can be presented to help students grasp these components. Whatever the focus of discussion, however, there must be a "conceptually adequate" definition that demonstrates the prevailing attributes of the concept and its scope of application.

Case studies can be an important strategy to help students grasp the concept, but it is important not to fall into the trap of "model cases." Model cases, as noted previously, can place inappropriate boundaries on a concept and cause the individual learning the concept to assume too narrow a scope of application. The learner may reach the conclusion that, if such an example is a model, then *all* instances of the concept will appear to be similar. Even relatively clear-cut concepts, such as *Mobility*, have numerous variations related to arthritis, postoperative ambulation, amputation, and many more instances, in addition to the positive aspects such as athleticism. Focusing on a model case of *Mobility*, perhaps in the case of a distance runner who clearly is very "mobile," will present an unnecessary and unrealistic example that does not show the range of use of the concept and its relevance in numerous instances in nursing. Another example is *Asepsis*, which is closely related to the concepts of *Sepsis* and *Infection*, either of which can be found along a continuum ranging from simple, localized infection to systemic septic shock and intractable conditions. Exemplars, presented from a variety of perspectives and showing the concept in numerous contexts, will help students grasp not only the defining characteristics of the concept but the many ways in which it can be used appropriately.

Summary

Methods of concept development, particularly concept analysis and clarification, are essential in a concept-based curriculum. Following a documented approach to clarification can help ensure that the appropriate components of a concept are understood well, presented clearly, and described in relevant contexts similar to how students are expected to use the concepts. Essential components of a concept, which are sufficient to provide a high degree of clarity, can be articulated within a concept development framework. This can provide a structure for presentation and discussion, as well as for making sure that all critical aspects are addressed. It is important, however, that the approach to analysis and clarification be one that promotes critical thinking, relevant application, and a strong grasp of the concept as demonstrated by the students' ability to use the concept effectively (Rodgers, 2000). Presenting concepts from a philosophical perspective that acknowledges conceptual change and helps students actively engage in that process through evaluation of the usefulness and effectiveness of concepts can promote not only concept learning but the spirit of inquiry, adaptability, and ongoing evaluation that is essential to effective nursing practice and growth.

REFERENCES

Bissonnette JB: Adherence. In Giddens JF, editor: *Concepts for nursing practice*, St. Louis, MO, 2013, Mosby, pp 50–57.

Buchanan L: Stress. In Giddens JF, editor: *Concepts for nursing practice*, St. Louis, MO, 2013, Mosby, pp 280–290.

Fehr B: Prototype analysis of the concepts of love and commitment, *Journal of Personality and Social Psychology* 55:557–579, 1988.

Giddens J, Edds K: Coping. In Giddens JF, editor: *Concepts for nursing practice*, St. Louis, MO, 2013, Mosby, pp 291–298.

Morse MM: Exploring the theoretical basis of nursing knowledge using advanced techniques of concept analysis, *Advances in Nursing Science* 17(3):31–46, 1995.

Morse JM, Mitcham C, Hupcey JE, Tason MC: Criteria for concept evaluation, *Journal of Advanced Nursing* 24:385–390, 1996.

Norris CM: *Concept clarification in nursing*, Rockville, MD, 1982, Aspen.

Oxford Dictionary of English (2nd Ed. Rev). Oxford, 2005, Oxford University.

Rodgers BL: Concepts, analysis, and the development of nursing knowledge: The evolutionary cycle, *Journal of Advanced Nursing* 14:330–335, 1989.

Rodgers BL: Concept analysis: An evolutionary view. In Rodgers BL, Knafl KA, editors: *Concept development in nursing: Foundations, techniques, and applications*, 2nd Ed, Philadelphia, PA, 2000, W. B. Saunders, pp 77–102.

Rodgers BL, Cowles KV: The concept of grief: An evolutionary perspective. In Rodgers BL, Knafl KA, editors: *Concept development in nursing: Foundations, techniques, and applications*, 2nd Ed, Philadelphia, PA, 2000, W. B. Saunders, pp 103–117.

Schwartz-Barcott D, Kim HS: A hybrid model for concept development. In Chinn PL, editor: *Nursing Research Methodology: Issues and Implementation*, Rockville, MD, 1986, Aspen, pp 91–101.

Walker LO, Avant KC: *Strategies for theory construction in nursing*, Norwalk, CT, 1983, Appleton-Century-Crofts.

Walker LO, Avant KC: *Strategies for theory construction in nursing*, 5th Ed, Upper Saddle River, NJ, 2011, Pearson Education.

Wilson J: *Thinking with concepts*, London, 1963, Cambridge University Press.

Developing a Concept-Based Curriculum

4

Jean Giddens

Curriculum development, regardless of the discipline, the type of learning program, or the level of learner, follows a general and predictable process. In academic institutions, faculty members are responsible for the development, implementation, and evaluation of the curriculum. A curriculum should reflect and support the overarching goals of the academic institution and nursing school. Nurse educators must also consider changes in professional nursing standards, health care trends, higher education, and the general society when undertaking curriculum work. Special interest groups, stakeholders, and a number of policy, regulatory, and political variables must also be addressed. Needless to say, curriculum work is a complex process that requires many resources. Several books have been written that describe curriculum development and revision in detail; such detail is beyond the scope of this chapter. The intent of this chapter is to provide a general overview of curriculum development as a frame of reference, and then focus on unique elements associated with curriculum development when a conceptual approach is planned.

Overview Of The Curriculum Development Process

The term *curriculum* refers to the arrangement of content within courses that form an academic program of study. The purpose of a curriculum is to provide an organizational structure to the academic program so that learners can successfully achieve predetermined outcomes. In many cases, nursing schools or departments offer multiple programs, and thus multiple curricula are used—one to support each program.

Curriculum work is not a one-time event, but rather a continuous process. As Figure 4-1 shows, a new curriculum or a curriculum revision occurs based on evidence that changes must be made. After a curriculum revision committee develops or revises a curriculum, faculty and institutional approval must be gained before it is implemented. Implementation of the curriculum occurs with a clearly identified plan to evaluate program outcomes and assess student learning. Data are regularly collected and analyzed by faculty, which in turn provides evidence for curriculum changes as they are needed.

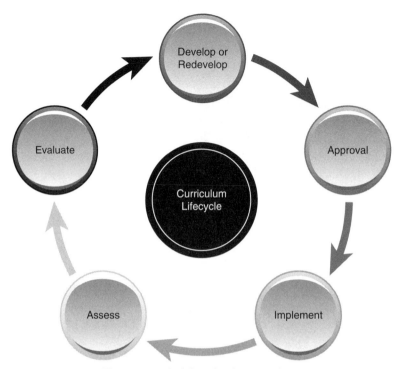

Figure 4-1 The life cycle of a curriculum.

Internal and External Context for Curriculum Change

Although it is often said that faculty "own" the curriculum, several internal and external forces and issues play a significant role in the curriculum. Nurse educators must maintain an ongoing awareness of these contextual factors. Internal factors include expertise of the faculty in curriculum development, other curricula offered by a nursing school or department, institutional policies, institutional culture, student characteristics, physical resources, and human resources (e.g., the number of faculty, staff, and students enrolled). Professional practice standards, accreditation standards, regulatory bodies, and clinical agencies are examples of external drivers of change that have policy implications. Other external factors include the characteristics of the community served (such as population demographics and culture), socioeconomic factors, health care access, explosion of technology, and employer demand.

Mission, Vision, and Philosophy

As a starting point for curriculum development, faculty should consider the institutional mission and vision statements of the parent institution as well as those stated by the nursing school or department. A mission statement explains

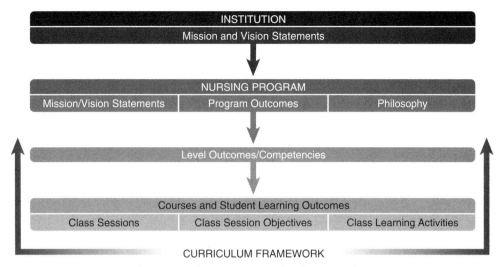

Figure 4-2 Elements associated with a curriculum.

organizational purpose or meaning; better stated, the mission statement describes why an entity exists. A vision is a statement of what an entity wants to be or what it wishes to accomplish. Thus mission and vision statements serve as a compass for the parent institution, as well as the nursing school or department. Consistency and clear linkages between the nursing school mission and the institutional mission and vision statements are required (Figure 4-2).

A school's philosophy is a statement of values or beliefs held collectively by the faculty, providing consistency and integrity to all curriculum elements (Csokasy, 2002). These values and beliefs guide faculty in actions and decision-making related to curriculum and academic delivery. Developing a philosophical statement is very time consuming and difficult. As a result, many schools have moved away from developing formal philosophical statements. As this movement has occurred, a greater emphasis has been placed on having a well–thought-out organizational framework.

Planning Curriculum Outcomes and Competencies

Another central element of curriculum development is identification of curriculum outcomes and competencies. Outcomes and competencies (two related but different educational terms) are used to describe learning gained by students within the program and are based on professional standards. A competency is a general statement that describes the knowledge, skills, and behaviors necessary for students to successfully perform in a professional context. A learning outcome is a specific statement that describes what a student will be able to do in a measurable way. Multiple outcomes may be written for each competency.

During the past 15 years, there has been growing trend in higher education for increased emphasis on student outcomes (learning outcomes and competencies) as a result of completing a curriculum. Curriculum goals and outcomes are not new, but the expectation of being able to measure and track students' accomplishment of outcomes certainly has increased with the assessment movement. The increased emphasis on outcomes is higher education's response to the public's expectation for accountability (Boland, 2004). The need to track outcomes, coupled with advancements in technology, has resulted in the development of applications specifically designed for outcome measurement and tracking of student learning outcomes.

There are different levels of learning outcomes and competencies. End-of-program outcomes (also referred to as program learning outcomes) and competencies are the "terminal" or "end points" that serve as the expected characteristics of graduates as a result of completing the program (Whittmann-Price and Fasolka, 2010). As a matter of sequence, faculty should consider identifying the program outcomes and competencies after addressing the mission, vision, and philosophy and before identifying the organizational framework.

In addition to program outcomes, there is a need for "markers" at specified points within the curriculum to assess students' progress while in a program. These markers, known as "level outcomes" or "level competencies," are statements of the knowledge, skills, and attitudes expected of students and are typically written from a behavioral perspective in one of three domains (cognitive, psychomotor, or affective). Typically there are sequential components to a competency requiring development over time, hence the need for competencies at various stages or levels within the curriculum. In a concept-based curriculum, competencies link to concepts. Learning outcomes and competency statements drive assessment of student learning within the curriculum and thus serve as the structural foundation of program evaluation. For this reason, it is critical these components link clearly throughout the curriculum.

Curriculum Design: Developing an Organizational Framework for the Curriculum

An organizational framework is essentially the blueprint or design of a curriculum, helping to clarify the scope of content and how it will fit together. It provides a mental picture of how the curricular elements interface with the curriculum approach. The organizational framework is driven by the mission and vision statements and, to a lesser extent, by the philosophy statement. There are a number of organizational frameworks for nursing curricula from the "traditional" approach (i.e., the Tyler curriculum model widely in use since 1950) to eclectic and nontraditional approaches. The trend in nursing education has been away from traditional curriculum approaches toward nontraditional approaches. A concept-based curriculum is an example of a nontraditional approach.

The process of developing the organizational framework includes identifying and defining the structural elements (e.g., themes, principles, threads, competencies, and/or concepts) to gain a shared understanding about what these elements mean. In addition, developing a clear vision and message about how the curriculum elements link together is critical. These elements must be constructed so that program outcomes and competencies are achievable.

Course Design

Courses within a curriculum should reflect the program learning outcomes and level competencies. In other words, individual courses within a curriculum should be logically structured to facilitate students' achievement of the level competencies and program learning outcomes. For this reason, level competencies are used as a basis for course development.

Expectations of student learning within courses are written as course learning outcomes (or in some cases, course competencies). Course learning outcomes are more specific and concrete than level competencies; these outcomes not only provide the foundation for course development but also for assessment of student learning within the course. Clear linkages between course learning outcomes and level competencies help to ensure curricular cohesion; in a concept-based curriculum, the outcomes should link to concepts. Student learning outcomes have gradually replaced the behavioral objectives approach historically used in higher education. An ongoing debate about the use of objectives, student learning outcomes, and competencies has been reflected in the nursing education literature for more than a decade (Bastable, 2013; Caputi, 2010; Goudreau et al., 2009; Nelson, Howell, Larson, & Karpiuk, 2001; Whittmann-Price & Fasolka, 2010). Regardless of the decisions made by a faculty to use student learning outcomes, competencies, or objectives at the course level, the most important point is that they provide clarity about the content focus and expectations of students.

The development of the course takes shape by developing a syllabus. Specific elements for course development include determining the type of course (e.g., lab, clinical, seminar, or didactic), the course description, student learning outcomes for the course, the number of academic credits, course delivery, a course outline (i.e., delineation of specific topics/content featured within the course), and planned strategies for teaching, learning, and evaluation. Teaching, learning, and evaluation strategies should align with the student learning outcomes, and the type of course. Arrangement and sequencing of the courses collectively should be considered to ensure continuity, consistency, and balance. Such a process occurs regardless of the curriculum design.

Curriculum Model

A visual model of the curricular framework shows the association between the concepts and elements within the curriculum. This can help faculty and students to gain a better understanding the curriculum. Boland (2012) advises a "less is more" principle related to the development of curricular models, warning that too complex of a model leads faculty to "spend more time trying to interpret and understand the framework than they do actually implementing and evaluating it" (Boland, 2012, p. 144).

Curriculum Evaluation

Curriculum evaluation is an organized and ongoing appraisal of the curriculum to determine strengths and weaknesses. It should include all curriculum elements and professional standards, as well as the success of the students and graduates of the program. Planning the evaluation of a curriculum occurs as a part of curriculum development, and continues during and after implementation. A strong evaluation plan involves having a clear understanding of the evaluation standards and type of data to collect, a consistent data collection process, and a clear plan for data analysis. Curricular improvements should be data driven, as a result of this process.

As mentioned previously, program outcomes, level competencies, and student learning outcomes at the course level provide the infrastructure for an evaluation plan. Data should be collected at the course level, at markers along the way, and at the end of the program using a variety of data collection methods. Data sources can include students, faculty, employers, preceptors, nurses, and curriculum and course documents.

Developing a Curriculum Using the Conceptual Approach

Educators interested in developing a concept-based curriculum follow a similar process described in the previous section. This section will take each of the steps and describe in greater detail unique elements when developing a curriculum using a conceptual approach.

Internal and External Context for Curriculum Change

The same contextual factors previously described apply to a concept-based curriculum and there are a few other factors to be aware of. One of the most important internal contexts to consider is faculty expertise related to the conceptual approach. Expertise is needed for appropriate decision-making and to clearly articulate the conceptual approach to administrators, other faculty, students, and external stakeholders. This expertise is also needed to address resistance.

External factors especially important to consider when adopting a conceptual approach are the perspectives of the employers and nurses within the community. It is essential that this group of stakeholders understand why the curriculum is changing and how it is envisioned; eliciting their support and input is critical. Most employers welcome a change in the education system, especially if it means that the nursing graduates will have higher-level thinking and problem-solving skills. Communicating the competencies of graduates is important for prospective employers. Nurses in the community, particularly those who interface directly or indirectly with students, must have an understanding of the changes that will occur, especially with regard to clinical education. Most nurses welcome a change in the educational system if it means that clinical education is less burdensome to the practice areas and if their input is solicited.

Mission, Vision, and Philosophy

Faculty adopting a concept-based curriculum should consider the institutional mission and vision statements of the parent institution as well as those stated by the nursing school or department—an expectation consistent with any curriculum development process. It is possible that the conceptual approach will influence a revision of the nursing school's mission, vision, and/or philosophy statement, although it is also possible these statements can remain unchanged.

Curriculum Outcomes and Competencies

After the mission and vision have been considered, curriculum committees usually develop or revise the program learning outcomes (end of program outcomes) and level competencies. These outcomes and competencies often are sequenced before the curriculum design because the curriculum outcomes serve as a beacon or directional endpoint. Faculty often ask how the program learning outcomes should be stated for a concept-based curriculum. As mentioned previously, the curriculum design is essentially a blueprint or design of the curriculum and is driven by the mission, vision, and program learning outcomes; in other words, it is not the program learning outcomes that are different, but rather the way the curriculum is packaged. For example, a common program outcome of an undergraduate curriculum may read something like this:

> *Collaborate as a member of an interdisciplinary team to improve the quality of health care.*

Such an outcome or competency is a desired expectation of any nursing graduate from any nursing program regardless of the type of curricular design of the nursing program. However, the curricular design is the vehicle faculty choose to ensure that students can achieve this learning outcome. Thus, there is little difference in this process, although the design should be taken into account to ensure that the structure fits the identified outcomes and competencies.

Developing a Design for a Concept-Based Curriculum

One of the truly unique hallmarks of developing a concept-based curriculum is with the design. As mentioned previously, curriculum design is an organizational framework—or better stated, the blueprint for the curriculum. This process includes selecting and defining the concepts and determining how the concepts will be linked together within the curriculum. Figure 4-3 shows these general steps.

Concept Categories

Once the decision to adopt a concept-based curriculum is made, there is a tendency for faculty to immediately begin identifying and negotiating concepts to be included. However, a step that ideally precedes this process is the identification and development of concept categories. Concept categories provide structure to the curriculum through the organization of concepts and provide greater clarity about what the concepts represent. Development of the concept category involves establishing criteria or parameters regarding how concepts for each category are selected, identified, and applied. Parameters establish the rules or criteria involved in determining if a concept fits within a category and also provide some guidelines regarding how it is framed and eventually taught. If a large number of concepts fit within a broad category, subcategories (or macroconcepts) are useful for further organization. The number and type of concept categories used within a curriculum can vary considerably and is one of the ways a curriculum from one school can distinguish itself from another. Three common concept categories are presented and described as examples in the following sections.

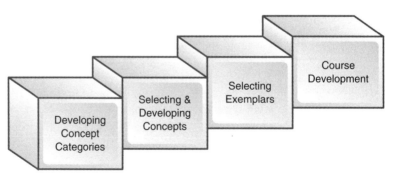

Figure 4-3 Critical steps for concept-based curriculum design.

Health and Illness Concepts

Health and illness concepts represent a patient's health status in relationship to three general goals of health care: the promotion of health, the prevention of disease, and the treatment of illness. These goals are interrelated and often thought of in terms of functional processes. An established categorical description used to determine if a concept fits in the category might be something as simple as "*A physiological or psychosocial health response.*" Concepts such as *Gas Exchange, Infection, Mobility, Immunity, Cognition,* and *Mood* clearly fit, while concepts such as *Delegation, Policy,* and *Ethics* clearly do not. Health and illness concepts should be considered from three contexts: *health continuum, life span continuum,* and *environment of care.* These contexts serve as guiding principles related to how the concepts are selected, presented, and applied (Figure 4-4).

For example, the concept *Immunity* represents conditions across the health-illness continuum (health promotion, acute illness, and chronic conditions) and across the life span continuum (infants, children, adolescents, adults, and older adults), and care delivery occurs across multiple environments (within hospital units and clinics, and from a community health perspective, public health perspective, and global perspective). Parameters such as these help with the selection process, and provide clarity for use within the curriculum.

Because the health and illness concept category is very large, macroconcepts help to further organize concepts. For example, a curriculum committee may wish to use a macroconcept such as Oxygenation and Homeostasis as a category for *Perfusion, Gas Exchange,* and *Clotting.* Likewise, the concepts *Infection, Mobility,* and *Tissue Integrity* logically fit under the macroconcept Protection and Movement (Table 4-1). Concepts organized within a macroconcept tend to be closely interrelated.

Professional Nursing Concepts

Concepts that represent the critical attributes and collectively describe professional nursing practice are referred to as professional nursing concepts. These concepts are associated with professional comportment—or in other words, these concepts link with the identity of nursing as a health care profession. Many of these concepts actually link more broadly to desired behaviors of all health care providers. Concepts such as *Professionalism, Ethics, Collaboration,* and *Patient Education* all clearly fit in a category such as this.

Established parameters for the Professional Nursing Concept Category can be presented from the context of the *individual nurse,* the *unit of care,* and from a *system perspective* (see Figure 4-4). For example, a concept such as *Policy* could

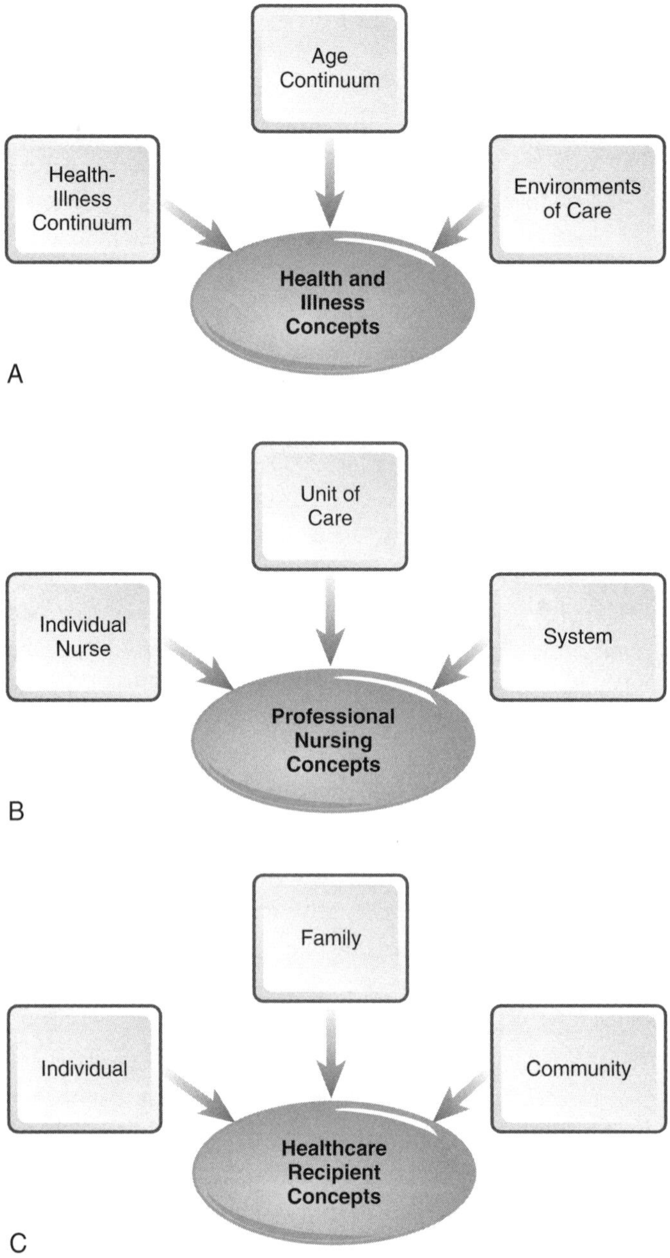

Figure 4-4 Concept categories and parameters. **A,** Health and illness concepts. **B,** Professional nursing concepts. **C,** Health care recipient concepts.

TABLE 4-1 **Examples of Macroconcepts and Concepts Within the Health and Illness Concept Category**

CONCEPT CATEGORY	MACRO-CONCEPT	CONCEPTS
Health and Illness Concepts	Coping and Stress Tolerance	Stress
		Coping
	Oxygenation and Homeostasis	Perfusion
		Gas Exchange
		Clotting
	Emotion	Mood
		Affect
	Protection and Movement	Immunity
		Inflammation
		Mobility
		Tissue Integrity
	Regulation	Cellular Regulation
		Thermoregulation
		Glucose Regulation
		Intracranial Regulation
		Acid-Base Balance
		Fluid and Electrolyte Balance
		Nutrition
		Elimination
	Cognitive Function	Cognition
		Psychosis
	Maladaptive Behavior	Addiction
		Interpersonal Violence
	Sexuality and Reproduction	Sexuality
		Reproduction

be presented from the context of how policies affect a nurse in direct care (such as a uniform policy or a policy regarding central line care), how policies affect an organization (such as admission policies and reimbursement policies), and how policies affect the health care system. This concept could also be presented by taking one specific policy such as the Health Insurance Portability and Accountability Act and framing it from the context of the individual nurse, the organization, and the health care system.

Professional nursing concepts can be further organized with macroconcepts. For example, *Health Care Organizations, Health Care Economics, Health Policy,* and *Health Care Law* logically are grouped under the macroconcept *Health Care Infrastructure*. Likewise, the concepts *Care Coordination, Caregiving,* and *Palliation* logically fit under the macroconcept *Health Care Delivery* (Table 4-2).

TABLE 4-2 **Examples of Macroconcepts and Concepts within the Professional Nursing Concepts Category**

CONCEPT CATEGORY	MACRO-CONCEPT	CONCEPTS
Professional Nursing Concepts	Health Care Delivery	Care Coordination Caregiving Palliation
	Health Care Infrastructures	Health Care Organizations Health Care Economics Health Policy Health Care Law
	Care Competencies	Communication Collaboration Health Care Quality Safety Technology and Informatics Evidence
	Attributes and Roles	Professionalism Clinical Judgment Leadership Ethics Patient Education Health Promotion

Health Care Recipient Concepts

The health care delivery system has made major strides, particularly during the past two decades, to move from a disease-centered perspective (in which the health care providers controlled all aspects of care) to a patient-centered model whereby recipients of care are not only informed of care options but are partners in the care decisions. Delivery of patient-centered care requires the recognition that health care recipients are very diverse, and thus health care decisions must take into account the unique needs and preferences of the patient (Institute of Medicine [IOM], 2001).

As a concept category, health care recipient concepts—also known as patient profile concepts—represent the unique and distinct attributes of all health care recipients. It is essential for nurses to understand these fundamental concepts for the successful delivery of patient-centered care. For organizational purposes, it may be useful to use the macroconcepts *Personal Preferences* and *Attributes and Resources* to further categorize concepts in this category (Table 4-3).

Health care recipient concepts should be considered from three contexts: the *individual,* the *family,* and the *community* (with community care ranging from a local to a global perspective). These contexts serve as guiding principles related to

TABLE 4-3 Examples of Macroconcepts and Concepts Within the Health Care Recipient Category

CONCEPT CATEGORY	MACRO-CONCEPT	CONCEPTS
Health Care Recipient	Attributes	Development
		Functional Ability
		Family Dynamics
	Personal Preferences	Culture
		Spirituality
		Motivation
		Adherence

BOX 4-1 Hallmarks of "Good" or Well Chosen Concepts for Nursing Education Curricula

- The concept represents an important group of conditions or situations (exemplars) encountered in nursing practice.
- The concept has application across multiple courses and contexts within the curriculum.
- The concept is useful to the learner.
- The concept can be used logically and consistently by all faculty.

how the concepts are selected, presented, and applied (see Figure 4-4). For example, the concept *Culture* represents the shared attitudes, beliefs, traditions, norms, values, and preferences of individuals and groups of people. Culture should be considered when providing care to an individual health care recipient, and it should be considered in the context of that individual's family members—recognizing that there may be value conflict between the two. Culture from the perspective of community has applications for example, when doing work in public health nursing and when setting health policy. Context parameters such as these (the individual, the family, and the community) help with the selection process, and provide clarity for use within the curriculum.

Selecting and Identifying Concepts

Selecting concepts generally follows after or in conjunction with determining concept categories. Oftentimes, faculty will have ideas about certain concepts that should be included, and thus the formation of larger categories as concepts are discussed is natural. One of the biggest challenges, however, is determining how many and which concepts to include. The hallmarks of "good" or well-chosen concepts to include in a nursing curriculum are presented in Box 4-1. Typically, the concepts should be very familiar and understandable to nursing faculty because they represent the scope of nursing practice. If there is a lot of confusion among faculty about a proposed concept, it should be critically analyzed to determine if it represents a concept associated with a specialty (a microconcept) or if it really represents a larger category of concepts (a macroconcept). Distinctions between microconcepts and macroconcepts are presented in Chapter 1.

Because concepts should be reflective of contemporary nursing and health care practice, an examination of the nursing and other health sciences literature is helpful. Another strategy is to review the list of concepts included in other concept-based curricula. A recent study involving a survey of 10 nursing programs or consortiums using a concept-based curriculum identified a total of 54 benchmark concepts—in other words, those that were most prevalent among reporting schools (Table 4-4). This study validated that although most concept-based curricula have similar featured concepts, there is not a single "correct" list. In other words, one should expect some variability in the concepts if comparing concept-based curricula across a number of schools (Giddens, Wright, & Gray, 2012).

As concepts are recommended and negotiated, a consistent, systematic selection process should be applied to determine if a concept is "accepted" or "rejected" for final inclusion in a curriculum. Five questions that link back to the hallmarks of a "good" concept can be used to facilitate such a process:

1. Does the concept represent an important group of conditions or situations (exemplars) encountered in nursing practice?
2. Can the concept be applied across multiple courses and contexts within the curriculum?
3. Is the concept useful to the learner? In other words, will the learner find a clear application of the concept to the courses and clinical experiences?
4. Can the concept be used logically and consistently by all faculty?
5. Is the concept sustainable? In other words, is this a concept that will be applicable in 10 years?

Another element associated with concept selection is clearly defining and developing the concept. It is critical that faculty have a shared understanding of the concept— meaning how it is defined, what it represents, how it is applied, and how it will be taught. It is recommended that a template be followed so this work progresses consistently. The template may vary depending on the type of concept category, because one template does not necessarily work for all categories. A sample template for health and illness concepts and a template that works for professional nursing concept categories and health care recipient concepts are provided in Boxes 4-2 and 4-3, respectively.

TABLE 4-4 Common Concepts Used in Concept-Based Nursing Curricula		
ATTRIBUTE CONCEPTS	**PROFESSIONAL NURSING CONCEPTS**	**HEALTH AND ILLNESS CONCEPTS**
Advocacy	Caring	Addiction
Culture	Clinical Judgment/Critical Thinking	Anxiety
Development	Collaboration	Cognition
Diversity	Communication	Grief
Family	Educator	Interpersonal Relationships
Spirituality	Ethics	Mood
	Evidence	Self
	Health Care Delivery	Stress/Coping
	Economics	Violence
	Law	Acid Base
	Quality	Cellular Regulation
	Policy	Behavior
	Health Promotion	Elimination
	Leadership	Fluid and Electrolyte
	Patent Centered	Gas Exchange
	Professionalism	Immunity
	Safety	Infection
	Technology/Informatics	Inflammation
		Intracranial Regulation
		Metabolism
		Mobility
		Nutrition
		Pain/Comfort
		Perfusion
		Reproduction
		Sensory Perception
		Sexuality
		Sleep–Rest
		Thermoregulation
		Tissue Integrity

Data from Giddens J, Wright M, Gray I. (2012). Selecting concepts for a concept-based curriculum: Application of a benchmark approach. *Journal of Nursing Education, 51*(9):511-515.

Selecting Exemplars

Exemplars provide clinical context for the concept. Exemplars—or "examples"—are necessary for deep conceptual learning because they provide a specific situation for the broader, more abstract concept. Conceptual learning holds limited value unless students can anchor what they have learned to specific examples. From this perspective, this is where traditional nursing content fits in a concept-based curriculum. However, in a concept-based curriculum, exemplars are carefully selected to minimize excessive curricular content. It is not uncommon for nursing faculty to be initially skeptical about limiting the number of exemplars.

BOX 4-2 **Sample Template for Health and Illness Concepts**

- Definition
- Scope, Type, or Category(s)
- Individual Risk Factors and Populations at Risk
- Physiologic Process and Consequences
- Assessment
  - History
  - Examination
  - Diagnostic Studies
- Clinical Management
  - Primary Prevention
  - Secondary Prevention (Screening)
  - Collaborative Interventions
- Interrelated Concepts

BOX 4-3 **Sample Template for Professional Nursing Concepts and Health Care Recipient Concepts**

- Definition
- Scope, Type, or Category(s)
- Attributes
- Theoretical Links
- Context to Nursing and Health Care
- Interrelated Concepts

The value of managing excessive curriculum content is based on the premise that when students gain a deep understanding of a concept, they are able to make connections from the concept to other exemplars—even ones they have not been formally taught in the classroom. It is also important to remember that students will be exposed to far more exemplars in the clinical setting when providing care to patients and families. Thus, an essential part of the concept-based curriculum is capitalizing on students' exposure to exemplars that are not formally taught in the didactic courses and helping students make purposeful cognitive connections.

Setting a process for exemplar selection helps to reduce the temptation to include exemplars that happen to be a favorite topic of one or more faculty, which tends to lead to a curriculum pitfall of excessive content. Ideally, data-driven decisions are made to select exemplars. When data driven decisions are made, students will be exposed to the most important and prevalent content. In other words, faculty will focus on the most common things the student will see in practice. Health and illness concepts are best selected on the basis of state, national, and global health incidence and prevalence statistics (such as the Centers for Disease Control and Prevention), although there may be an occasional situation where an exemplar is selected because it has unique value in illustrating the concept. Exemplars for professional nursing concepts and health care recipient attributes are best identified by current literature and contemporary events, although some events that are more historic may have particular value if they have forever influenced nursing and/or health care practice today.

Another challenge when selecting exemplars is that most exemplars link to multiple concepts; thus, there is risk for duplication of content within the curriculum. For example, the exemplar pneumonia logically links to *Infection*, *Gas Exchange*, *Fatigue*, and *Fluid and Electrolyte Balance*—but it is completely unnecessary to teach it four times as an exemplar of four concepts! A curriculum plan or map should be developed that clearly shows exemplars used for each concept. When teaching a specific exemplar, the lesson plan should include time for students to reflect on concepts that are interrelated with the exemplar.

Didactic Courses and Course Development

The next major step in concept-based curriculum design is the development of courses that feature concepts and conceptual learning. Course learning outcomes are a starting point for course development. Unlike program outcomes that are not strikingly different in a concept-based curriculum compared with other curricular structures, course learning outcomes are different. They should clearly emphasize the application of concepts within the course and must link to the program learning outcomes. Earlier in this chapter the following example of a program learning outcome was provided:

> *Collaborate as a member of an interdisciplinary team to improve the quality of health care.*

An example of a course learning outcome that might be developed within a concept-based curriculum follows:

> *Analyze the concept of Quality as a foundational element of health care delivery.*

Notice that this learning outcome specifically addresses the concept and clearly links to the program learning outcomes. More detail regarding writing learning outcomes is presented in Chapter 7.

Many additional variables influence the direction of the curriculum when considering course design. First, the type of degree offered drives the total number of credit hours; thus the number of credits for nursing courses will vary. Also, the institution may influence some of the courses offered and the sequencing of those courses. The semester that students are admitted to the nursing program (e.g., direct entry, entry after 1 year, or entry after 2 years) must also be considered. Finally, the prerequisites and corequisites influence what is considered primary content or review content. For example, if anatomy, physiology, and pathophysiology are prerequisite courses taken before entry into the nursing curriculum, the courses designed for conceptual teaching will look different than if information from these courses were to be integrated into the nursing courses. After those things are considered, a decision must be made about how the concepts will be used within the courses. Two common paths may be taken: integrated into traditional population-focused and topic-focused courses, or as concept-focused courses.

Integration Into Population-Focused and Topic-Focused Courses

For years, nursing curricula have arranged content around population (such as pediatric, maternal child, adult, and geriatrics) and topic areas (such as mental health, leadership, and community). When this approach is used for a concept-based curriculum, concepts serve as a common link between and among courses. For example, all of the health and illness concepts apply to all population groups and thus are the core organizers of content for these courses. The focus for the concept presentation and exemplars are based on the population-specific elements for that concept. Professional nursing concepts fit into many of the fundamentals and leadership-type courses. In this approach, clinical courses continue to be closely linked to the traditional population-focused didactic courses.

One advantage to the population-focused and topic-focused approach is that many of the courses and clinical experiences maintain a level of familiarity and may be more readily accepted by faculty. A drawback to this approach is that faculty are tempted to change very little and claim they teach the concepts while continuing to overload students with content. Also, there is the potential for each faculty member in each course to teach the concept overview, which would result in duplication of effort.

 Misconceptions and Clarifications

| **Misconception:** A simple way to develop a concept-based curriculum is to identify major concepts within courses of an existing curriculum. | **Clarification:** Designing a concept-based curriculum does not occur by simply identifying concepts in an existing curriculum, nor does it occur by adding concepts to an existing curriculum (i.e., an "add-on" approach). In concept-based curricula, concepts provide the structural framework for courses and content. Courses are redesigned with a specific plan for integration of concepts within the concepts. |

Concept-Focused Courses

The other approach is to develop concept-focused courses that feature an integration of population groups. Courses typically follow the identified concept categories (Table 4-5). For example, there may be a series of courses that feature health and illness concepts, a series of courses that feature professional nursing concepts, and a course that features health care recipient concepts. If macroconcepts are identified within concept categories, these may also be useful to consider so that concepts that are closely related are taught in a similar course.

When a concept-focused course approach is used, concepts and the dedicated exemplars are featured once in the designated didactic course. Thereafter the concepts are presented as interrelated concepts. Conceptual links across population groups and types of settings are made. Clinical courses should be designed to follow concept courses, and should apply concepts from *all* courses (health and illness, professional nursing concepts, and health care recipient concepts) into the clinical experience. In other words, clinical education represents the application and synthesis of all concepts, not just one group of concepts, in a variety of clinical sites and working with a variety of patient populations.

The benefit to this approach is that the concept is presented in greater depth, allowing for a deeper understanding to occur through exemplar reinforcement. However, this approach is not without challenges. It requires a very different teaching expectation among faculty and may result in the need for team teaching in the didactic courses. For example, the concept of *Gas Exchange* may be easy enough to teach, but the exemplars are likely to be representative of the health conditions across the age span, such as asthma in children and pneumonia in older adults. This approach also de-emphasizes specialty content, and thus it is important that

---

TABLE 4-5 Sample of Course Arrangement in a Concept-Based Curriculum for a Four-Semester Nursing Program

SEMESTER 1	**SEMESTER 2**
Nursing Skills and Assessment Lab	Health and Illness Concepts 1I
Patient Attributes Concepts	Professional Nursing Concepts I
Health and Illness Concepts I	Evidence-Based Nursing Practice
Clinical Practicum I	Clinical Practicum II
SEMESTER 3	**SEMESTER 4**
Health and Illness Concepts III	Global Health
Professional Nursing Concepts II	Concept Synthesis
Clinical Practicum III	Clinical Practicum V
Clinical Practicum IV	Capstone

students have varied clinical experiences so they have clinical exposure across populations and specialties.

In addition to concept-featured courses, consideration of other types of courses should be included. As an example, a fundamentals course that teaches basic nursing skills and health assessment skills may still be necessary. In a baccalaureate curriculum, faculty may wish to offer a separate course focusing on community-based nursing, public health nursing, or nursing research. When this is the case, applicable core concepts are still to be woven into these courses.

Clinical Courses

Decisions about design of clinical courses are just as important as didactic course decisions. The conceptual approach offers an opportunity to break away from the traditional clinical education model that has been in place for well over 50 years. The emphasis has historically been placed on inpatient clinical courses that focus on caring for an assigned patient or patients, mimicking the work assignments of staff nurses in a designated clinical focus area. Students typically go to the unit to meet their assigned patient, review the medical record, and prepare required clinical paperwork prior to their clinical experience. During the clinical day, students receive report and care for their assigned patient(s), which may include the following activities: hygiene care, toileting, activity and exercise patient assessment, nutrition and dietary needs, medication administration, and a number of other interventions ordered by the physician. For many care activities, direct supervision by the nursing instructor or a primary nurse is required. Throughout the program, the advancement of clinical expertise is measured by the number and/or complexity of the patients assigned, and the gradual increase in competence and independence demonstrated by the student in the provision of care. Although this "patient of the day" approach still holds value, there are some clear downsides, including a tendency for students to focus on tasks and considerable downtime experienced by students as they wait for the necessary supervision (by an instructor or primary nurse) to complete nursing intervention (such as a dressing change or administering a medication). This type of clinical learning should be considered one teaching strategy among many other strategies used for clinical education.

Clinical courses designed for a concept-based curriculum include a variety of learning opportunities for students to apply several concepts in a number of ways and in a number of clinical situations. Clinical courses should link to didactic courses in that the application of concepts from the corequisite didactic courses should be emphasized. The learning activities can vary from the standard "patient of the day" to a multitude of "concept-focused" learning within the clinical area. As an example, students might be assigned to study the concepts of *Immunity,*

Inflammation, and *Infection* within a designated group of patients, and also consider how the concepts of *Health Policy* and *Health Care Economics* apply to the patient situations. Learning focuses on comparing and contrasting evidence of positive or ineffective immune status and evidence of or risk for inflammation and infection (among multiple patients) and includes the reinforcement of previously learned or new exemplars representing those concepts. Students might be asked to review policies that impact the care, as well as to compare health payment plans of the patients they are caring for. Simulation, with an emphasis on specified concepts, is another type of clinical learning activity that is effective. (Additional examples of concept-based teaching strategies for clinical education are presented in Chapter 6.)

Students should still have clinical experiences and exposure to various population groups and settings (e.g., pediatrics, adults, geriatrics, mental health, intensive care, and community) but with less emphasis placed on marching all students through the exact same set of clinical experiences. For example, in some programs offering concept-based curriculum, students have an opportunity to choose the clinical courses (known as clinical intensives) that appeal to them after completing foundational clinical courses. Thus, in a given semester, students in the same cohort are applying concepts from the didactic concept courses in different clinical areas. Such an approach allows greater flexibility and efficiency in the way clinical sites are used (Giddens et al, 2008).

Tips For Success: Developing and Implementing the Concept-Based Curriculum

Most faculty are aware of the significant effort associated with developing and implementing a new curriculum. This section offers specific tips for enhancing success.

Expect a Range of Emotions

The reaction and emotions expressed among faculty will range from being thrilled about the change to being angry. Occasionally, opposing faculty may be disruptive to the work. Supporting faculty may become concerned if they are unable to gain full consensus among the faculty. Although this would be ideal, in most cases it is unrealistic. It is important that support for the curriculum work reaches *critical mass* to move forward, and energy should be directed toward working with those who seek change.

Managing Resistance

Any new curriculum (especially a concept-based curriculum) represents significant effort from the curriculum committee and for faculty assigned to teach new courses. This can be threatening because nurse educators are forced to step out of their teaching comfort zone. Resistance to change is a natural reaction (particularly when the proposed change is not universally or well-understood). Anticipating and accepting resistance as a normal part of the process is helpful so that strategies can be developed to ensure forward movement. Resistance is usually put forth by one or more strongly vested faculty who defend the old curriculum. Common arguments against change (presented below) can be easily countered by using nonadversarial responses.

"We Have Always Done It This Way! Why Should We Change?"

Extensive changes in health care, coupled with a growing call for change, makes this argument easy to address. Two early reports from the IOM, *Crossing the Quality Chasm* (IOM, 2001) and *Health Professions Education* (IOM, 2003), call for improvements to be made in health sciences education to improve quality of care. Specifically, several competencies such as patient-centered care, evidence-based medicine, working as part of an interdisciplinary team, focusing on quality improvement, and using information technology were emphasized, along with the need to address changing student demographics and teaching using active learning strategies (IOM, 2003). More recently, one of four key messages in the *Future of Nursing* report (IOM, 2010) is the need for nurses to achieve higher levels of education through *an improved education system* that promotes seamless academic progression. Another landmark publication, *Educating Nurses* (Benner, 2010), also describes the need for radical transformation of the education of nurses. A focus on and delivery of content in the traditional way does little to prepare nurses for the "situated cognition and action" needed for clinical practice (Benner, 2010, p. 13). Although these reports do not specify that a conceptual approach is needed, they all emphasize the need for an improved education system for effective health care delivery. In other words, the traditional approach to nursing education is outdated and is no longer preparing nurses adequately for the current health care system. It is simply the professional and ethical obligation of a higher-education professional to address and embrace this call for critical change within the nursing profession.

"Our NCLEX Pass Rates Are Good"

One of the biggest barriers to innovative curriculum work is the justifiable fear of reduced first-time pass rates on the National Council Licensure Examination (NCLEX). For years, first-time NCLEX pass rates have unofficially served as the gold standard measure of the quality of a nursing program. The Boards of Nursing in all states closely monitor first-time pass rates, setting a minimum standard expected of schools—which in some cases may create additional concern. In truth, the first-time NCLEX pass rate is only one indicator of program quality considered by accreditors. Other important measures include student and program measures. Examples of student measures include evidence of achievement of program outcomes, competencies, and student learning outcomes within courses, time to graduation, graduation rates, and the diversity of student enrollment. Program measures include an adequate number of qualified full-time faculty for the program(s) offered; tracking, orientation, and evaluation of preceptors and adjunct faculty; integrity of the curriculum; and a systematic approach to curriculum evaluation. The point is, a nursing program can have excellent first-time pass rates and yet can fail to address the changing needs of the nursing workforce. There is no intent to suggest that concept-based curricula will increase first-time pass rates, but no evidence exists that programs with a concept-based curriculum have a lower pass rate. In fact, according to a survey of 57 nursing programs offering a concept-based curriculum, 35% reported higher first-time pass rates, 42% reported no changes in first-time pass rates, and 5% reported lower first time pass rates. Eighteen percent of respondents did not know the impact on first-time pass rates (many had not yet graduated students from their new concept-based curriculum (Sportsman, 2013).

"What Evidence Proves the Conceptual Approach Is Better?"

It is interesting that this question is raised over and over again, especially when there is plenty of evidence that our traditional approaches to educating the health care workforce have not been effective for the changing health care environment (Benner, 2010; IOM, 2001, 2003, 2010). One can defend the traditional approach by citing "evidence" based on first-time NCLEX pass rates, as though this is the only evidence that counts. Although there is no "proof" that a conceptual approach for nursing education is better, the education discipline has plenty of evidence regarding improvements in learning and improvements in content management when the conceptual approach is applied (Ambrose et al., 2010; Erikson, 2002; Erikson, 2008; Schmidt, McKnight, & Raizen, 1997; Sousa, 2010; Zull, 2002). Over time, as more nurse educators adopt the conceptual approach, we can expect the availability of published program and student learning outcomes.

"Our Faculty Workloads Are Too Heavy"

The nationwide faculty shortage has several implications for nursing programs, but what is especially problematic is the effect on faculty work assignments. It is unlikely that any nursing program has faculty who are not concerned about the amount of work associated with their jobs. Thus, this is a statement and argument that is universally heard with any project, initiative, or change introduced to faculty groups. Adopting the conceptual approach does require significant effort, not only in the development of the curricula, but also in the change of teaching.

However, an expectation of all faculty, regardless of the type of institution or type of discipline, is maintaining currency in educational delivery. Curriculum development and advancing one's teaching should not be presented as an "add-on" or "additional work"—rather, this should be presented as a professional obligation to the students, institution, and profession. Further, once the curriculum is developed and faculty begin the process of transitioning their teaching practice, there is often a level of energy and excitement that is associated with the teaching-learning process. Over time, once faculty learn how to effectively teach conceptually, they are likely to experience teaching effort that is more effective and efficient.

Secure Resources

Undertaking any major effort is met with greater acceptance if adequate resources are available. Examples of helpful resources include:

- Expert consultation from nursing faculty experienced in the development of a concept-based curriculum and or consultation from faculty in other disciplines, such as education
- Site visits to nursing programs that have successfully adopted a concept-based curriculum
- A dedicated work assignment for key faculty who are leading the curriculum change
- Faculty development opportunities, especially in the area of concept-based teaching and learning
- Support from senior administrators in the nursing program, particularly for additional help needed and/or flexibility in teaching assignments, admissions, and course scheduling as the new curriculum is rolled out

Expect Hard Work and Encourage and Support One Another

Curriculum redesign is very challenging work that takes a great deal of time. Faculty should not begin with an expectation that the process will be completed quickly. A great deal of discussion, negotiating, and reflection is needed at the beginning of the process to elicit input and build the initial support needed to begin work, let alone the numerous meetings and work needed for the actual curriculum design. Developing a trusting, encouraging, and supportive relationship among the faculty—particularly those directly involved in the curriculum work—helps to sustain the effort needed over time.

Engage Your Clinical Partners

Collaborating with nurses in practice settings (particularly those from clinical agencies where students complete clinical experiences) in the development and implementation of the curriculum can enrich the work and deepen the relationships between the nursing school and the clinical agency. Eliciting input and support from these important stakeholders during the process increases the level of acceptance of the planned changes. This is particularly important when redesigning clinical education and attempting to implement significantly different learning activities within the various clinical sites.

Summary

This chapter has reviewed the general steps associated with the development of a concept-based curriculum. Some of the most important points to reiterate about this process include:

1. The general curriculum development process is the same—it is the curriculum design that is unique
2. Concepts used for the curriculum represent concepts of nursing practice as opposed to concepts representing the discipline of nursing from a theoretical perspective
3. Content saturation is avoided by carefully considering the concepts and the number of exemplars to include in the curriculum
4. Course design (including clinical course design) and teaching practices will change
5. The process is difficult and often is met with resistance. The resistance met is not a reason to abandon the idea but rather represents a difference in the values and perspectives of faculty. The lack of understanding related to the conceptual approach is often the greatest source of resistance.

REFERENCES

Ambrose SA, Bridges MW, DiPietro M, Lovett MC, Norman MK: *How learning works. 7 Research-based principles for smart teaching*, San Francisco, CA, 2010, John Wiley & Sons.

Bastable S: *Nurse as educator*, 4th ed., Sudbury, MA, 2013, Jones & Bartlett.

Benner P, Sutphen M, Leonard V, Day L: *Educating nurses: A call for radical transformation*, San Francisco, CA, 2010, Josey-Bass.

Boland DL: Developing curriculum: Frameworks, outcomes and competencies. In Billings D, Halstead J, editors: *Teaching in Nursing*, 4th ed., St. Louis, MO, 2012, Elsevier.

Boland DL: Program evaluation and public accountability. In Oermann M, Heinrich K, editors: *Annual Review of Nursing Education*, New York, NY, 2004, Springer.

Caputi L: Curriculum design and development. In Caputi L, editor: *Teaching Nursing: The Art and Science*, Volume 1, 2nd ed, Chicago, IL, 2010, College of DuPage.

Csokasy J: A congruent curriculum: Philosophical integrity from philosophy to outcomes, *Journal of Nursing Education* 41:469–470, 2002.

Erikson L: *Concept-based curriculum and instruction*, Thousand Oaks, CA, 2002, Corwin Press.

Erikson L: *Stirring the head, heart, and soul. Redefining curriculum, instruction, and concept-based learning*, Thousand Oaks, CA, 2008, Corwin Press.

Giddens J, Brady D, Brown P, Wright M, Smith D, Harris J: A new curriculum for a new era of nursing education, *Nursing Education Perspectives* 29(4):200–204, 2008.

Giddens J, Wright M, Gray I: Selecting concepts for a concept-based curriculum: Application of a benchmark approach, *Journal of Nursing Education* 51(9):511–515, 2012.

Goudreau J, Pepin J, Dubois S, Boyer L, Larue C, Legault A: A second generation of the competency-based approach to nursing education, *International Journal of Nursing Education Scholarship* 6(1), 2009.

Institute of Medicine: *Crossing the quality chasm*, Washington, DC, 2001, National Academies Press.

Institute of Medicine: *Health professions education*, Washington, DC, 2003, National Academies Press.

Institute of Medicine: *Future of nursing*, Washington, DC, 2010, National Academies Press.

Nelson ML, Howell JK, Larson JC, Karpiuk KL: Student outcomes of the healing web: Evaluation of a transformative model for nursing education, *Journal of Nursing Education* 40(9):404–413, 2001.

Schmidt WH, McKnight CC, Raizen S: *A splintered vision: An investigation of U.S. Science and mathematics education. U.S. National Research Center for the Third International Mathematics and Science Study (TIMSS)*, Dordrecht, Netherlands, 1997, Kluwer Academic Publishers.

Sousa DA: *Mind, brain, and education. Neuroscience implications for the classroom*, Bloomington, IL, 2010, Solution Tree Press.

Sportsman S, for the Academic Consulting Group: *Nationwide concept based curriculum survey analysis [PowerPoint presentation]*, Amsterdam, 2013, Elsevier.

Whittmann-Price RA, Fasolka BJ: Objectives and outcomes: The fundamental difference, *Nursing Education Perspectives* 31(4):233–236, 2010.

Zull JE: *The art of the changing brain*, Sterling, VA, 2002, Stylus Publishing.

Conceptual Learning 5

Jean Giddens

A key challenge shared among all instructors—regardless of the discipline or student level—is creating an optimal platform for learning. In higher education, faculty are primarily hired because of their expertise in their respective discipline and often lack an understanding of how people learn. Faculty tend to focus on honing a teaching style that works well for them with little thought how student learning occurs as a result of their efforts. A common assumption held by new and many seasoned instructors is that students learn as a result of attending a class or completing a course. The flaw in this thinking is nested in a general lack of understanding about what learning is and the science behind learning. The truth is, learning is not something that is "done" to students by instructors; rather, learning is something that students accomplish themselves. Instructors have a role in facilitating this process by creating purposeful and engaging learning activities in an optimal learning environment.

Conceptual learning was identified in Chapter 1 as one of five separate but interrelated elements associated with the conceptual approach. The desired outcome associated with conceptual learning is that students gain a deep understanding of concepts and the ability to transfer ideas to other situations through cognitive connections. Nurse educators adopting the conceptual approach are usually eager to learn how to teach conceptually. However, gaining an understanding of the science of learning is foundational to teaching. Put another way, the science of instruction builds on the science of learning. Having an understanding about how learning occurs must precede conversations about best teaching practices. In this chapter, principles associated with the science of learning will be presented, along with the linkages to the conceptual approach.

Definition of Learning

There are a large number and wide variations in learning definitions. Ambrose and colleagues offer a contemporary definition reflective of the science of learning.

They define learning as "a *process* that leads to *change* which occurs as a result of *experience* and increases the potential for improved performance and future learning" (Ambrose, Bridges, Dipietro, Lovett, & Norman, 2010, p. 3). Emphasis on the words "process," "change," and "experience" represent three key components of the definition. *Process* is emphasized because learning is a brain-based physiological process that occurs in the mind. Learning cannot be directly seen or measured, but inferences that learning has occurred are made based on student performance. *Change* is emphasized because learning results in a change in students' knowledge, beliefs, behaviors, attitudes, and values. Although the change occurs over time, an enduring impact occurs. *Experience* is emphasized because learning is shaped by the interpretation and response to former and current experiences. In any given situation, students may or may not be aware of the influence of experiences on their learning. These key components become clearer in the sections that follow.

Educational Neuroscience: How The Brain Learns

Learning is a complex process with multiple variables. During the past few decades, there has been increasing interest in *educational neuroscience*, a term used to describe the interrelationship between neuroscience, teaching practices, and psychology as key components of the learning process (Figure 5-1). It is imperative

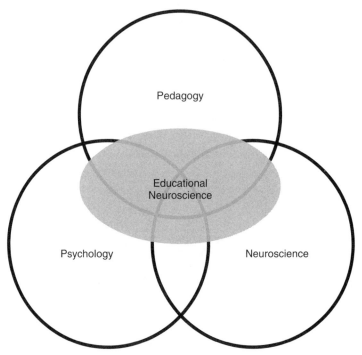

Figure 5-1 Educational neuroscience represents pedagogy, neuroscience, and psychology.

that all educators gain an understanding of these components in order to fully grasp how to effectively facilitate conceptual learning. In the sections that follow, a very brief review of brain structures and function is included as a foundation for understanding the process of learning. The discussion of brain function is only done with the intent to explain how the brain learns.

General Brain Function

A very simplistic summarization of what the brain does can be described in three words: *sensing*, *integrating*, and *responding*. **Sensing** refers to an ongoing process whereby the brain takes in data signals (input) from a variety of internal (physiologic) and external (environmental) sources. **Integrating** is the process of sorting and grouping data and then making sense of those data. Put another way, integration is the process of recognition and interpretation that occurs with the sum of all the data signals (Zull, 2002). **Responding** refers to the outcome of the data integration. The brain sends information to target areas, triggering a wide variety of physiologic responses, including regulatory and motor responses (voluntary and automatic movements). The transfer of data signals—from sensory input, integration, to a motor response—is continuous, cyclic, and automatic; sensory input triggers integrative activity, which triggers motor activity (Figure 5-2).

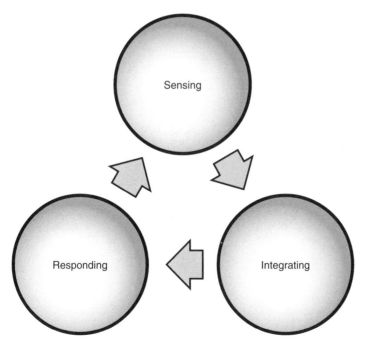

Figure 5-2 Sensing, integrating, and responding are ongoing and continuous processes within the brain.

Brain Structures

The brain is a highly complex structure within the central nervous system and is composed of three major units: the cerebrum, the brainstem, and the cerebellum. The cerebrum comprises the largest part of the human brain and is divided into two hemispheres (right and left), each of which are divided into four lobes (frontal, temporal, parietal, and occipital) as shown in Figure 5-3. The outer layer covering the cerebrum is the cortex; together, these are referred to as the *cerebral cortex*. Neurons within the cortex are responsible for many of the highly sophisticated aspects of cognitive functioning. The limbic system is a group of structures that connect higher and lower brain functions (Figure 5-4). Together these structures regulate emotion, mood, pleasure, and motivation. Box 5-1 presents a review of limbic structure functions. The brainstem, located at the base of the brain, includes the midbrain, pons, and medulla. The cerebellum, tucked behind the brainstem and beneath the occipital lobe of the cerebrum, coordinates movement and equilibrium (see Figure 5-3).

Neurons

At the cellular level, neurons are built for efficiency in transmitting information. Neurons have three functional characteristics: (1) generate nerve

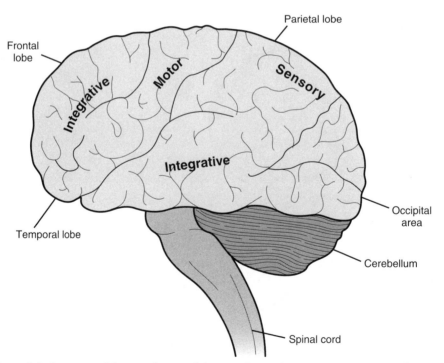

Figure 5-3 Structures of the outer brain and functional areas for sensory, integrative, and motor functions.

impulses, (2) transmit nerve impulse to other parts of the cell, and (3) transmit signals to other cells and organs to create an effect. Neurons direct signals from cell to cell through dendrites and axons. Axons of one cell extend to the dendrites of the next cell (Figure 5-5). Signals are sent back and forth from cell to cell across the synapse, the gap between axons and dendrites. The process is

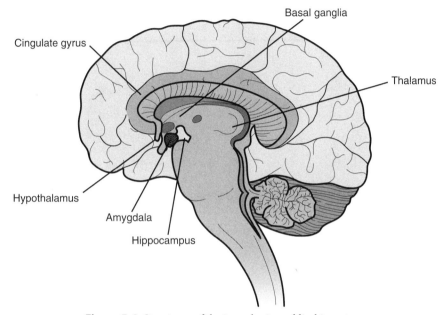

Figure 5-4 Structures of the inner brain and limbic system.

BOX 5-1 **Limbic Structure Functions**

- The *basal ganglia* are paired structures that are involved with automatic and voluntary movement.
- The *thalamus* is a relay center and transfers nearly all signals to the cerebral cortex.
- The *hypothalamus* regulates the autonomic nervous system and the endocrine system.
- The *amygdala* is a walnut-sized structure that influences emotional states on sensory input and has a role in determining what memories retained. This structure has tremendous influence on learning.
- The *hippocampus* plays a significant role in information transfer to long-term memory.
- The *cingulate gyrus* serves as a message transfer channel to and from the limbic system.

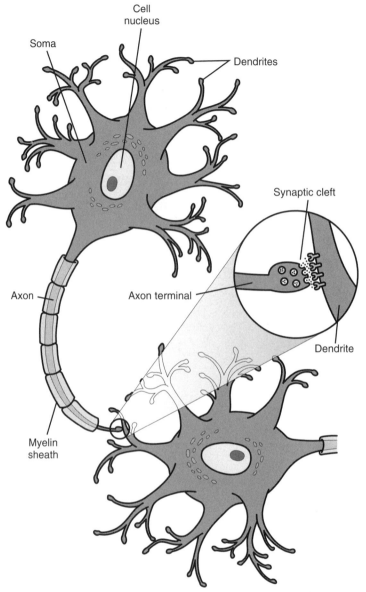

Figure 5-5 Structure of a neuron. (Dustin Hull Heuston, PhD, "Structure of a Neuron" [figure], *The Third Source: A Message of Hope for Education*, with James W. Parkinson [Salt Lake City, Utah: printed by author, 2011], 235.)

enhanced by the myelin sheath—a coating over the axon and neurotransmitters. It is estimated that the human brain has more than 100 billion neurons, with as many as 10,000 connections per neuron! Connections become a very important point in the next section when considering the brain structures related to learning.

Brain Structures and Learning

Obviously the brain is far more complex in its function and structure than the preceding discussion would suggest. However, this simplified approach (sensing, integrating, and responding) provides a useful framework for understanding the science of learning because the same process supports learning. The primary activity of human learning involves taking data in, integrating the data for meaning, and responding. These functions occur through trillions of data signals and networks between the neurons within the cerebral cortex.

Various areas of the cerebral cortex play specific roles in the process of sensing, integrating, and responding as it relates to learning. The function of sensing involves receiving auditory, visual, olfactory, and tactile data signals. The thalamus, located at the base of the cerebrum, serves as the brain's primary dispatch center for sensory data. It sends data signals (which are essentially nothing more than isolated bits of data) to the temporal and frontal regions of the cerebral cortex for integration. The integrative process involves merging these data into clusters that become meaningful, such as visual recognition, language, and images. These meanings are further integrated in various ways that become thoughts, ideas, and plans for action (Zull, 2002).

Considering the physiologic function of various areas of the cerebrum, this process makes a great deal of sense. The frontal lobe is responsible for memory retention, higher level cognitive function, expressive speech, and voluntary eye and motor movement, while the temporal lobe controls receptive speech and the integration of visual, somatic and auditory data. Interpretation of spatial data information occurs within the sensory cortex of the parietal lobe, while the processing of visual data occurs in the occipital lobe.

"Responding" refers to carrying out the action plans formed in the integration phase. Located centrally within the cerebrum are the paired basal ganglia, which are responsible for the initiation, execution, and completion of voluntary and automatic movement. These muscle movements are necessary for a variety of actions, from blinking, swallowing, running, scratching, and—more specifically related to learning—the formation of speech and the ability to write, draw, and perform other related movements. The transfer of data signals (sensory input, integration, and motor response) is continuous and cyclic; sensory input triggers integrative activity, which triggers motor activity. The motor activity in turn serves as sensory data that start the cycle again. This cycle is automatic, and to a large extent it is subconscious. Figure 5-6 shows the pattern and flow of sensory input, data integration, and motor response across the brain.

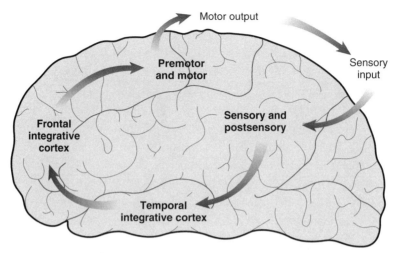

Figure 5-6 Sensory input, data integration, and motor response. (Modified from Zull JE: *The art of changing the brain: enriching the practice of teaching by exploring the biology of learning.* Sterling, VA, 2002, Stylus Publishing, LLC.)

The Learning Brain

Sensing, Integrating, and Responding

Learning involves a combination of taking in new information and active thinking to translate that information into meaning and appropriate actions. The three elements of sensing, integrating, and responding once again apply to this discussion.

In a learning situation, new information presents as auditory, visual, olfactory, and tactile data signals. The intake of information from the sensing brain has limited benefit or use unless the information is applied. In other words, there must be a process whereby the student not only receives knowledge but also uses the knowledge in a way that requires the brain to actively integrate the information so it can be transformed into understanding and meaning. Little is gained in situations where there is an intake of new information without using that information to stimulate thinking, create ideas, or generate an action plan.

Based on the preceding discussion, it should be obvious that integration of information is a necessary step for learning to take place. Referring back to the previous section, two areas of the brain are involved with integration. The temporal integrative cortex involves memory of places and stories and information as facts. When new information comes in, the learner builds on existing knowledge – through existing neuronal networks. The frontal integrative cortex involves active mental energy, decisions, choice, and creativity. For this reason, learning is enhanced when there is balance between the two integrative sections. The outcome of a balanced approach is the transformation of a learner from a receiver of information to a producer of ideas (Zull, 2002).

Extending Neural Connections

The term *neuroplasticity* is used to describe the brain's ability to reorganize and restructure itself through the formation of new neural connections as a result of experiences (Dragansk & Gaser, 2004). Neuroplasticity is an outcome of effective learning. When the brain is challenged with new information and problem solving, the integrative process of the mind involves clustering of data. In other words, the brain forms patterns for meaningful organization and categorization of the information. New knowledge and information is matched to memory, extending neural networks. This process facilitates the construction and extension of neuron connections; new knowledge structures are built with a new baseline for incoming information.

Variables Influencing Learning

Emotion

It has been noted several times throughout this chapter that sensing is one of the primary functions of the brain. As noted earlier, sensing involves the input of information. The limbic system, particularly the amygdala, plays a powerful role in learning. Emotion influences the way sensory data are filtered. A positive emotional state favors conduction through the amygdala, and as a result, information reaches the integrative areas of the brain. Positive states also enhance memory retention, particularly when there is something novel about the learning activity. These effects have been shown through neuroimaging studies (Pawlak, Margarinos, Melchor, McEwen, & Strickland, 2003). In times of stress, fear, or anger, sensory data are largely sent to the lower-level reactive brain and data are not available for higher cognitive processing (Willis, 2010). This mechanism explains why it is very difficult to focus and learn in times of extreme stress and why individuals are more likely to be productive and learn when they are in a positive state. The amygdala also has a powerful effect in committing emotionally charged events (both positive and negative) to long-term memory. This phenomenon can be better understood by recalling a very happy or very sad event in your life. Details of such events are often easy to recall, even decades later.

Dopamine

Another critical variable associated with learning is dopamine, a neurotransmitter that facilitates the transmission of signals between neurons in the brain. Dopamine produces pleasurable feelings and the amount of dopamine released is influenced by emotional states. An increased release of dopamine is triggered with positive experiences and a drop in dopamine release can occur with negative experiences (Willis, 2010). This is an important principle because of dopamine's influence on learning. Dopamine acts as a reward mechanism in the brain related to learning and enhances the brain's translation of the information to memory. The nucleus accumbens, a dopamine storage structure, has been shown to release more dopamine when learners get answers right (which in turn creates a pleasurable feeling). Likewise, less dopamine is released when learners make a mistake or get an answer wrong (Salamone & Correa, 2002). This reward occurs when the brain is challenged and successful when thinking about new information and solving new problems. Individuals with mastery in basic math would not get rewarded with increased dopamine release for correctly solving simple mathematical questions (such as $3 \times 5 = x$, or $12 + 6 = x$) because arriving at these answers does not represent a challenge. An individual is also not rewarded with dopamine when he or she attempts to solve a challenging problem and gets the answer wrong or is unable to make substantive progress. When there is no reward, motivation is reduced. Gee (2007) describes the power of this effect in the context of computer games with multiple levels that are increasingly challenging. The dopamine-enhanced pleasure of successfully achieving a level motivates the player to go on to the next, more challenging level.

Movement

Another variable that impacts learning is movement. It has been known for years that the brain is more active when the body is active and less active when the body is stationary (Sosa, 2010). Body movement increases the flow of blood to the brain, thereby increasing the delivery of oxygen and glucose to neurons. Movement also enhances the brain's access to long-term memory. Studies also have shown that increased brain mass, cognitive processing, and mood regulation are associated with exercise.

Nutrition

The link between proper nutrition and peak learning has been well documented. Optimal neurotransmission within the brain requires adequate hydration. A reduced hydrated state can lead to poor concentration, emotional changes, and reduced cognitive abilities, all of which have a negative impact on the ability to learn. Carbohydrates are the main source of fuel for the brain. The importance of healthy carbohydrate choices is based on the evidence that wide fluctuations in sugar levels hamper effective neurotransmission. An intake of an excessive amount of simple sugar triggers insulin release, which can cause drowsiness. In contrast, complex carbohydrates are associated with a slower breakdown and absorption of sugar, providing a steady release of fuel. Fats and proteins are needed to enhance healthy neurons, which in turn impacts neurotransmission.

Sleep

The sleep-deprived brain negatively impacts learning because of a lack of focus and attention. In this state, the brain has a reduced ability to take in (sense) data from learning situations. Furthermore, when a person is in a sleep-deprived state, neurons are unable to efficiently coordinate data impulses leading to impaired cognitive capacity. Sleep deprivation also impacts the brain's ability to store information into memory and memory recall. Committing something that has recently been learned to memory requires sleep—or, put another way, sleeping well the night after learning new information or a new skill is important for memory and future performance (Sosa, 2010). Memory consolidation (i.e., stabilization of a memory) takes place during sleep through the strengthening of neural connections. Although this process is poorly understood, it is thought that this process is linked to sleep waves during different phases of the sleep cycle. Memory recall (i.e., the ability to access something previous stored into memory) is also negatively impacted with insufficient sleep. Several other negative impacts of sleep deprivation are reported in the literature, including mood. Specific to learning, sleep-deprived students tend to have lower grades and are more likely to be depressed compared with their peers who get adequate sleep (Wolfson & Carskadon, 1998).

Conceptual Learning In The Nursing Discipline

Throughout this chapter, the discussion has focused on the science of learning without specific reference to conceptual learning. The science of learning provides substantial evidence related to the benefits of conceptual learning. It should be increasingly clear that the conceptual approach is an opportunity for nurse educators to adopt strategies that enhance student learning. Ideally, this approach benefits learners not only while they are enrolled in nursing programs but also gives them the skills to emerge as efficient life-long learners throughout their career.

The massive volume of new knowledge generated throughout our society has made it impossible for any education program in any discipline to "cover" all the information in an academic program. With a greater understanding of how the brain learns, nursing educators must emphasize *learning with understanding* as opposed to *remembering and repeating facts*. Adopting the conceptual approach transforms the nursing education environment from a passive, static state with limited emotion or engagement into a vibrant, active, and challenging state with enhanced learning as an outcome. Given the preceding discussion about learning science, the relevance of this approach should be clear.

Timpson and Bendel-Simso (1996) described conceptual learning as a process by which students learn to organize information into logical mental structures and become increasingly skilled at thinking. Conceptual learning necessitates the use of facts as opposed to a focus on facts. The use of facts should be within the application of information in a larger context. In nursing, learning experiences should ideally be placed in the context of a clinical situation and be purposeful—in other words, learners should clearly recognize the benefit of what they are learning and how it applies to the practice of nursing.

Conceptual Thinking and Expert Thinking

As noted previously, the brain builds a network of new neural connections during the learning process. The conceptual approach cultivates this process because the learner is making connections by actively thinking about the interrelationships of information to concepts and the interface of concepts across multiple situations and contexts. Patricia Benner's classic work *From Novice to Expert* (Benner, 1984) presented narratives describing thinking approaches among nurses across a spectrum of five stages of expertise: novice, advanced beginner, competent, proficient, and expert. Expert nurses, using their enormous background of experiences, have an accurate and intuitive grasp of situations and know how to respond, even in unique situations not previously encountered. This ability comes from well-honed cognitive skills—that is, the ability to focus on important data and recognize situations, synthesizing and analyzing the meaning of those data, and connecting this information to previous knowledge and experiences for an appropriate and seamless response. Bransford, Brown, and Cocking (2000) point out that only a subset of one's total knowledge applies to any particular problem. Experts possess a rich and large reservoir of knowledge connected and organized around important concepts. They also have the skill to retrieve the applicable and appropriate knowledge related to a presenting problem, which is referred to as *conditionalized knowledge*. A key element of conceptual learning is honing the skill of conditionalized knowledge retrieval for problem solving.

Novices, by comparison, tend to have knowledge arranged in a list-like, disconnected fashion. They are unable to effortlessly and accurately respond to complex problems because they lack contextual experience, are more likely to have rigid or rule-based understanding of information, and tend to approach problem solving from a linear-thinking approach. New graduates who lack conceptual thinking skills are challenged during the transition to practice because they lack not only depth in clinical experiences but also the cognitive skills needed to make conceptual connections.

Conceptual Learning and Meaningful Patterns

Conceptual organization allows an expert to see patterns and relationships not apparent to novice learners. Conceptual learning fosters the development of cognitive organization that is ultimately useful in specific contexts in which information is applicable, and it supports deep understanding. The organization of information into a conceptual framework allows for an enhanced ability to transfer and apply information to a new situation (Figure 5-7). The ability of the brain to transfer and apply information is hampered when knowledge lacks organization and presents as a set of disconnected facts. For this reason, a conceptual organization of information is foundational to clinical reasoning. The formation of clinical judgment and clinical reasoning in nursing requires an ability to make cognitive connections to past experiences and learn from new experiences, thus building the neural connections related to nursing expertise. Tanner's Model of Clinical Judgment (Tanner, 2006) presents this process as occurring from the perspective of noticing, interpreting, responding, and reflecting and doing so within situational context. The recognition of patterns related to specific conditions and situations is central to noticing and interpreting. This also closely links to the previous sections describing data intake and integrative processes within the brain. Responding represents the decision making and response that occurs in the brain. Reflecting, especially within the context of learning, represents the process of neuroplasticity (i.e., the formation of new neural connections within the brain as a result of experiences). Reflecting on these experiences drives deeper understanding for future learning.

Conceptual Approach and Deep Learning

Conceptual learning encourages students to focus on big ideas (or concepts) and apply information or knowledge to specific situations for context. Learning complex subject matter, such as nursing and health care, requires the ability to transfer what has been previously learned into problem solving activities in the context of

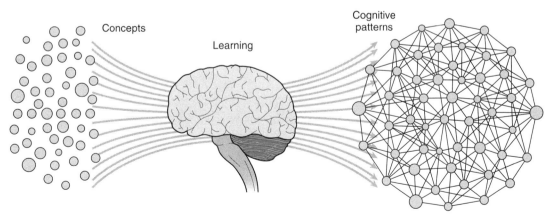

Figure 5-7 Conceptual learning is characterized by patterns and multiple linkages. (Based on "Knowledge Information," Idiagram, © Marshall Clemens; available at http://www.idiagram.com/ideas/knowledge_integration.html.)

> *BOX 5-2* **Exemplar: Conceptual Learning in Action**
>
> Reyna, a nursing student, is learning about the concept of inflammation. Prior to the class, she read a chapter on the topic. In class she listened to a 15-minute presentation by the instructor and then viewed a 5-minute video highlighting the physiologic response to inflammation. In her collaborative learning group, she shared a story about a time she experienced an inflammatory reaction and how her situation linked to what she just learned. Her group then completed a case study featuring a situation involving a patient with an inflammatory condition and reinforced risk factors, typical presentation, and collaborative interventions for the situation. The instructor led a discussion session about the case, posing specific questions to the learning groups, including the interrelationship of the concept of inflammation to other concepts. The class concluded with a short reflective writing activity in which Reyna wrote what she learned about her new understanding of the concept.

clinical situations. It does little good for students to learn about concepts in the absence of clinical examples, or exemplars. Benner and colleagues (2010) frame this from the position of integrative teaching practices—in other words, framing student learning of concepts and exemplars in the context of a patient situation or clinical problem. Conceptual learning, particularly when framed in a clinical context, engages the learner with an application of information to things that are clearly relevant. This engagement and active application of information facilitates understanding and commits this understanding to long-term memory (Box 5-2).

What Does All of This Mean for Nursing Faculty?

The preceding sections related to how the brain learns and conceptual learning underscore the need to rethink what is taught in nursing curricula and best practices for teaching. Superficial coverage of large volumes of nursing content must be replaced with a deep understanding of concepts. However, there must be a sufficient number of clinical examples (exemplars) to allow in-depth study; this is necessary to allow students to fully grasp the concept (Bransford et al., 2000). Connecting information to concepts over time further enhances this process, thus making the case for an established set of concepts to be used over a curriculum.

Teach With Balance

Traditionally, teaching has focused on delivering information in a student-passive approach. Assuming the students are paying attention, information is sent to the back portion of the cortex. The student must have an opportunity to integrate that information (using the frontal integrative cortex) to gain a deep and enduring understanding (Zull, 2002). Passive learning focusing on the memorization of facts is hard work because such an activity lacks context, and associations. It is just as problematic when students are exposed to learning activities without an infusion of information. Conceptual learning should be balanced with a focus on the concept. A combination of concrete experiences involving reflection and student-centered learning where students are involved in abstract thought, problem solving asking questions (thinking), hands-on activities, and activities requiring students to test their assumptions are central to conceptual learning. The application of such cognitive skills leads to more effective learning.

Misconceptions and Clarifications

Misconception: A student-centered learning activity is essentially the same as conceptual learning.

Clarification: Conceptual learning is enhanced with student-centered activities, but conceptual learning does not automatically occur simply by designing a student-centered learning activity. Optimal conceptual learning occurs when:

- Learners build on previous knowledge
- The learning activity focuses on a concept and is tied to the clinical context
- Students are fully engaged in the activity and perceive the learning activity as useful
- Reflection is used to facilitate deep connections
- The learning environment is safe

Purposeful Learning

Conceptual learning must have a purpose that is apparent to the learner. Students' perception of the value of what is being learned influences motivation, which in turn influences what and how they learn (Ambrose et al., 2010). Transferring previous knowledge to a new learning situation is enhanced by not only creating a situation where students see the value or direct relationship to their area of study and the implications of why it is important, but that they can see the benefit while they are learning.

Build on Existing Knowledge

Enhanced learning occurs when students can build on existing knowledge and apply new knowledge in purposeful ways. That the brain constructs new knowledge and understanding based on what a person already knows is an important principle that serves as a starting point for conceptual learning. It is also just as important for students to retrieve the necessary and appropriate knowledge to solve a problem. Preexisting knowledge should be considered as a starting point when creating conceptual learning activities. However, some learners have incomplete or inaccurate understandings, and this can interfere with new learning (Ambrose et al., 2010). For this reason, it is critical that learning be extended from a body of accurate information, which underscores the importance of assessing students' baseline understanding.

Purposeful Reflection

Reflecting on learning situations and experiences is one of the most important aspects of the conceptual approach and is a key to optimal learning in general. Reflection is a time to think about what has just happened in the learning situation and to actively contemplate things such as what was successful and what was not successful, how the situation differed from a previous situation, or how what was learned links to previously learned concepts. Faculty should build in reflection as part of conceptual teaching to optimize cognitive connections to concepts and clinical contexts.

Manage the Learning Environment

Conceptual learning requires deep and purposeful thinking, and thus the learning environment must be free from unnecessary distractions and stress. Faculty must consider the tone of the classroom and the emotional state of students. For example, it is not uncommon for first-semester nursing students to feel completely overwhelmed with the nursing school experience. Added to that may be feelings of inadequacy in a highly competitive cohort, along with personal stressors. Collectively these things matter and can impair learning. Elimination of unnecessary emotional stressors in the classroom or curriculum and creating an emotionally secure environment (one where learners feel respected by their teachers and free from potentially embarrassing situations) helps to moderate other stressors.

Emotion Matters

As in any learning situation, conceptual learning is optimized when learners are engaged and in a positive emotional state. Students do not typically become engaged when sitting and listening to a lecture. Therefore, nursing faculty are encouraged to teach using a variety of conceptual strategies that enhance learner engagement in pleasurable ways. The real trick is learning to foster an emotional connection to material as opposed to just making learning fun. Novel teaching strategies that enhance curiosity are effective as long as there is actual learning involved. Concepts taught using unfolding case studies (featuring characters familiar to the students) or standardized patients enhance a positive emotional connection (Shuster, Giddens, & Roerigh, 2011).

Summary

Educational neuroscience refers to the science of learning and includes the interrelationship between neuroscience, teaching practices, and psychology. The brain processes associated with learning include sensing, integrating, and responding. The brain's ability to learn is impacted by multiple factors such as emotion dopamine, sleep, nutrition, and movement. Best practices in education have shown that learning is most effective when students link to and apply previous knowledge to new situations. Conceptual learning directly applies such principles; students learn concepts as big ideas and apply these to multiple situations and contexts, resulting in neuroplasticity. Faculty can enhance conceptual learning by teaching with balance, managing the learning environment, creating emotionally engaging learning activities that are purposeful, and promoting focused reflection.

REFERENCES

Ambrose S, Bridges MW, Dipietro M, Lovett MC, Norman MK: *How learning works*, San Francisco, CA, 2010, Jossey-Bass.

Benner PB: *From novice to expert*, Menlo Park, CA, 1984, Addison Wesley.

Benner P, Sutphen M, Leonard V, et al.: *Educating nurses: a call for radical transformation*, San Francisco, CA, 2010, Jossey-Bass.

Bransford JD, Brown AL, Cocking RR: *How people learn: Brain, mind, experience, and school*, Washington, DC, 2000, National Academy Press.

Dragansk D, Gaser C: Neuroplasticity: Changes in grey matter induced by training, *Nature* 427(22):311–312, 2004.

Gee JP: *What video games have to teach is about learning and literacy*, New York, NY, 2007, Palgrave Macmillan.

Shuster G, Giddens J, Roerigh N: Emotional connection and integration: Dominant themes among undergraduate nursing students using a virtual community, *Journal of Nursing Education* 50(4): 222–225, 2011.

Pawlak R, Magarinos AM, Melchor J, McEwen B, Strickland S: Tissue plasminogen activator in the amygdala is critical for stress-induced anxiety-like behavior, *Nature Neuroscience* 6:168–174, 2003.

Salamone JD, Correa M: Motivational views of reinforcement: Implications for understanding the behavior functions of nucleus accumbens dopamine, *Behavioral Brain Research* 137:3–25, 2002.

Sosa D: How science met pedagogy. In Sosa D, editor: *Mind, brain, and education*, Bloomington, IL, 2010, Solution Tree Press.

Tanner CA: Thinking like a nurse: a research-based model of clinical judgment in nursing, *Journal of Nursing Education* 45(6):204–211, 2006.

Timpson WM, Bendel-Simso P: *Concepts and choices. Meeting the challenges in higher education*, Madison, WI, 1996, Magna Publications.

Willis J: The current impact of neuroscience on teaching and learning. In Sosa D, editor: *Mind, brain, and education*, Bloomington, IL, 2010, Solution Tree Press.

Wolfson A, Carskadon M: Sleep schedules and daytime functioning in adolescents, *Child Development* 69:875–887, 1998.

Zull JE: *The art of the changing brain*, Sterling, VA, 2002, Stylus.

Teaching Strategies for Classroom and Clinical Settings

6

Linda Caputi

This book has covered many aspects of the conceptual approach to nursing education. This chapter addresses implementation of a conceptual approach for teaching to enhance student learning. Because it is important to provide a theoretical basis for practice, the chapter begins with a discussion about cognitive frameworks and teaching. This context is then applied to the type of thinking used in nursing practice. The last and largest part of the chapter addresses the use of concept-based teaching strategies to teach students.

Cognitive Frameworks

Constructivist learning theory explains the nature of learning as a process through which learners create their own learning. Constructivists believe information can be constructed in many different ways. As faculty introduce new information, students either add that new information to their existing cognitive frameworks or construct a new framework (Schunk, 2012). Cognitive frameworks, also known as mental frameworks and schemata, help the learner organize and interpret information. Cognitive frameworks can also be seen as a way of looking at the elements that provide a framework for the implementation of the teaching/learning process (Caputi, 2010a). This is part of the *integrating process* discussed in Chapter 5 through which learners sort and group data and then make sense of those data, all of which occurs within their preexisting frameworks. The preexisting frameworks give meaning to incoming data. For example, when a nurse hears the phrase "2 by 4," the nurse processes that information as meaning a wound dressing. If the student has a background in construction, that phrase may take on a different meaning and confuse the uninformed student when it is used in a nursing context.

As learners build their cognitive frameworks in nursing, the process of integrating incoming information into an existing schema from a nursing perspective becomes automatic. Novices often do not have an established mental framework related to what they are learning in their nursing courses. The framework used by faculty to organize information has an impact on how students build cognitive frameworks in which to place and understand the information.

Linear Teaching and Cognitive Frameworks

Nursing faculty have traditionally taught with a linear approach organized around specific content. For example, faculty teaching a medical condition in an adult-health nursing course often use a body systems/disease approach that looks similar to the approach illustrated in Figure 6-1.

In this example, the disease is the major focus and is presented from the context of the primary body system affected. Anatomy, physiology, and pathophysiology are often discussed to frame the disease and may be repetitive information from prerequisite courses. Each disease has a list of risk factors, signs and symptoms, and laboratory/diagnostic studies included with a discussion on assessment. Medical treatment and nursing management are discussed, along with expected patient outcomes. Throughout the course and curriculum, other health conditions are organized in similar fashion, independent of each other, and often in the absence of a patient context or consideration of how the information applies to nursing practice. Subsequently, students memorize facts about each condition or content area and build discrete cognitive patterns that may look similar to those in Figure 6-2. Organizing information into categories that are not within a patient context and are structured around diseases, with nursing interventions representing just one of the pieces of information on the linear path, does little to provide relevance of the knowledge in practice situations. These frameworks are rather abstract, and students struggle to understand the relevance of all the parts (Benner, Sutphen, Leonard, & Day, 2010).

Conceptual Teaching and Cognitive Frameworks

In the conceptual approach, faculty teach students about the big ideas in nursing by framing nursing content within concepts. Three categories of concepts previously described in Chapter 4 (Professional Nursing and Health Care Concepts, Health and Illness Concepts, and Health Care Recipient Concepts) are used as the basis to organize teaching and learning. Not only is the focus on specific concepts, but the student makes purposeful linkages to interrelated concepts within all three concept categories. Learning is nested in a situational context—that is, within the practice of nursing (Figure 6-3).

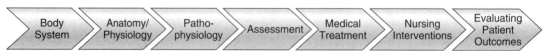

Figure 6-1 Body Systems Model for teaching nursing content.

Some of the same content that is taught in a traditional curriculum is presented, but it is presented as an exemplar of the concept rather than focusing on the condition or body system. Teaching using a conceptual organizing framework helps students

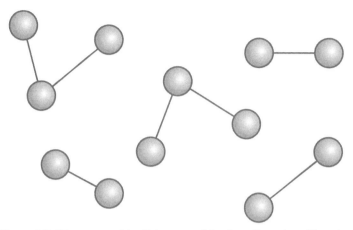

Figure 6-2 Discrete cognitive linkages resulting from linear-based learning.

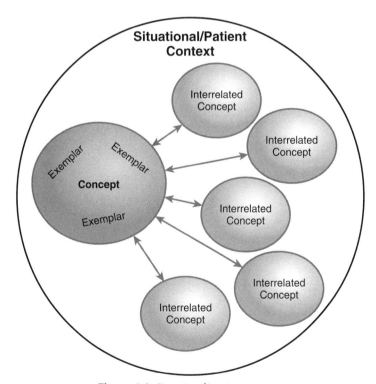

Figure 6-3 Situational/patient context.

develop cognitive patterns that look similar to the patterns shown in Figure 6-4. These cognitive skills facilitate transferability of information to other concepts and content.

Cognitive Frameworks and How a Nurse Thinks

Let's consider how a nurse thinks when approaching a patient. When the nurse knows the patient's presenting condition or medical diagnosis at the onset of care, the nurse's thinking may look something like that presented in Box 6-1.

Although the experienced nurse has an expectation about how the patient will present based on the medical diagnosis, many other aspects of the patient situation are assessed. According to Benner, Tanner, and Chesla (2009), the expert nurse has a deep understanding of the total situation and is able to focus immediately on salient aspects without wasting time and energy on a large range of alternative solutions. Thus the expert nurse takes in the whole picture of the patient. Although assessment related to the disease process is important, equally important are other salient aspects of the patient condition that are not related to the disease process. That is the type of thinking demonstrated in Box 6-1, and it represents many core nursing concepts.

This assessment often occurs before focusing on the medical condition. In fact, the medical condition may be near resolution and other issues may have developed that take priority. An example might be anxiety about a pending discharge, family issues, or an array of other problems. Nurses are able to deal with these concerns and problems because they think using concepts that are important to all of nursing practice, not just those related to the medical diagnosis.

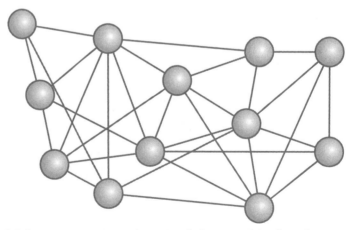

Figure 6-4 Pattern recognition and cognitive linkages resulting from the conceptual approach.

BOX 6-1 **The Thinking Nurse**

- Notice the patient's skin color and the concepts that skin color reflects (e.g., perfusion and oxygenation), which leads to an assessment of breathing characteristics and other related data; then consider laboratory test results, medications, and treatments related to these concepts.
- Consider how communication leads to an indication of cognition—the ability to process information.
- Consider anxiety and the concepts that anxiety reflects, such as pain, and then consider medication orders, treatments, and other concerns of the patient that may be causing the anxiety.
- Consider safety as it relates to the environment.
- Consider how tubes are related to hydration, output, and intravenous fluid orders.
- Consider care management and/or delegation.
- Consider how positioning is related to strength, mobility, and care management/delegation.
- Consider how visitors reflect family dynamics and the patient's support system.
- Consider other concepts, such as culture and functioning ability.

Teaching students from a medical model approach results in a greater emphasis on disease management and does not emphasize concepts within a nursing framework. When students who have been taught according to a medical model approach the patient, they begin their assessment by looking for signs and symptoms of the disease process as presented in their textbook. They might then evaluate the effect of treatments and look for evidence of complications. Students who have been educated with this focus on the medical condition and have built this type of cognitive framework must at some point in their practice assume a different perspective to better position themselves to engage in nursing, which deals with the patient's response to medical problems along with other health care concerns. Seeing the patient and nursing care from this perspective may not ever happen or may happen serendipitously.

Ideally, the patient's response to the medical problem is considered conceptually. The concepts addressed in Box 6-1 represent the patient's response to a medical problem but also the patient's response to many other health care issues. These findings represent the patient's responses, which are addressed by nurses. Many of these issues and concerns may be missed with a focus strictly on medical issues.

These considerations lead to the following questions: Would it not better serve students to teach them to think conceptually, using a concept-based cognitive framework rather than the medical model? If a concept-based cognitive framework is the focus of thinking we want students to use, how do we teach this way of thinking? It is critical that students be taught the concepts important to nursing practice and how they interrelate. In a concept-based curriculum, the major nursing concepts are taught with a focus on application within nursing practice. Nursing program content is presented based on patient situations that launch a cascade of relevant concepts, with the disease process the patient is experiencing just one issue related to the patient situation.

 ## Misconceptions and Clarifications

Misconception: One way to develop a concept-based curriculum is to take the current medical model curriculum, rename body systems as concepts (such as using the term "oxygenation" for the respiratory system), and then present the same information in the same manner as it was previously presented.

Clarification: Renaming body systems as concepts does not result in a concept-based curriculum. The curriculum is still organized around body systems and diseases. Although some health and illness concepts may relate to body systems, such as gas exchange, perfusion, nutrition, and others, in a concept-based curriculum, the content is organized in a different way and nursing is taught from a different perspective.

Conceptual Teaching and Cognitive Connections

The primary goal for faculty who are teaching nursing is to ensure that students learn how to use information the way the nurse uses it—that is, the student learns to think like a nurse. In the content-focused, body-systems approach to teaching, the risk is great that students will receive an excess of information that grows larger each year with the expanding knowledge base of nursing. This plethora of information, which has been determined to be essential for new nurses to learn, is overwhelming for students. Students tend to rely on memorization as the primary method of cognitive processing they use to meet their goal of passing the course. A concept-based approach to teaching provides students with experience in seeing patterns and using those patterns to think about the factual information they are learning. An overarching goal of the concept-based curriculum is to build conceptual understandings of nursing that are transferable to a variety of patient care situations. It is an approach that emphasizes *learning the processes of thinking* rather than memorizing a list of facts.

With a concept-based curriculum, faculty use teaching strategies that require students to look at nursing from the perspective of concepts important to nursing practice, coupled with active processing of information at the application and higher cognitive levels, to engage in thinking like a nurse. These teaching strategies are not hierarchical; that is, they do not build on each other and are not phased out and replaced with new strategies as the student progresses through the nursing courses. These strategies can be used in all nursing courses. The following simple example illustrates this point.

A patient with the diagnosis of anemia is assigned to a student. The student remembers the teacher explaining in class that a patient with anemia will have decreased hemoglobin. Using the medical model framework, the student attempts to recall other important information the teacher talked about when discussing anemia. The facts related to anemia are arranged as shown in Figure 6-1 and represent the student's primary thought processes.

On the other hand, a student who uses the conceptual learning framework also remembers that a patient with anemia has a decreased amount of hemoglobin, which results in decreased amounts of oxygen available to the body. The student then thinks about how concepts relate to the factual information about decreased oxygen, such as that decreased oxygen can result in decreased gas exchange and perfusion (both of which are concepts). The student then connects these concepts to attributes of the concepts that need to be explored, as well as to interrelated concepts. If the patient, for any reason, has decreased gas exchange and perfusion, what other concepts important to nursing practice and patient care may be interrelated? The answer may be:

- *Mobility*
- *Nutrition*
- *Anxiety*
- *Fatigue*

A patient assessment would confirm the presence of these interrelated concepts. The student would then look at the specific disease process related to the patient's anemia for further investigation. Understanding the specific pathophysiology of the anemia provides additional information for the nurse to investigate for this particular patient. Additionally, because teaching was presented conceptually, the student considers the following specific Health Care Recipient Concepts:

- *Development*
- *Culture*
- *Functional Ability*

These concepts are also investigated. Finally, the following concepts related to professional nursing and health care are linked:

- *Care Coordination*
- *Patient Teaching*

Decisions about delegation of activities such as ambulation and patient teaching are considered.

As demonstrated with this example, a person who thinks conceptually uses facts as a tool to determine patterns, connections, and deeper, transferable understandings.

Teaching these connections helps students make sense of the factual knowledge and teaches them to intuitively think in this manner.

Designing Classroom Learning Sessions

An important principle to remember is that teaching in a concept-based curriculum is not about teaching a list of concepts; rather, it is about *teaching students to think like a nurse* (Caputi, 2010b). What does this mean? How do nursing faculty conduct a classroom session to achieve conceptual learning as opposed to traditional learning in nursing? When teaching conceptually, keep these important principals in mind:

- Start with a formal concept overview or concept presentation.
- Teach designated exemplars for each concept.
- Link teaching to a patient or situational context.
- Link to preexisting understanding.
- Use a variety of student-centered teaching strategies for collaborative learning.

Concept Presentation

Each concept should be formally taught in depth (referred to as the *concept presentation*). The concept presentation should be incorporated within courses as part of curriculum planning. The sequencing of concept presentations is highly variable, depending on the curriculum design. Regardless of sequencing, faculty should develop a consistent approach to the concept presentation across all courses to enhance the development of students' expertise. Such a consistent approach is critical for curriculum integrity. A concept presentation includes many of the elements associated with a concept analysis, described in Chapter 3. The use of a standardized template to develop concept presentations is very helpful in achieving consistency. Table 6-1 is an example of a template that can be used to develop the concept presentation for Health and Illness Concepts. Table 6-2 is an example template for Professional Nursing and Heath Care Concepts and Health Care Recipient Concepts.

Once an outline of the concept presentation has been developed, faculty consider which learning activities to use for the concept presentation. As discussed in Chapter 5, learners benefit when a variety of teaching strategies are used. Developing a lesson plan for the concept presentation is helpful to create a balanced and purposeful learning experience for students. Table 6-3 shows an example of a lesson plan for a didactic classroom concept presentation for *Perfusion*.

Similar planning should occur for Professional Nursing Concepts and Health Care Recipient Concepts. Notice that the sample lesson plan represents

TABLE 6-1 **Concept Presentation Template for Health and Illness Concepts**

TOPIC	DESCRIPTION
Concept Definitions	A clear definition of the concept should be included so students (and faulty) are all working from a common definition; concept definitions can be easily found in the literature
Scope or Categories of Concept	All concepts have scopes or categories; a scope is like a continuum (such as hyperthermia, normothermia, or hypothermia), whereas categories are discrete distinctions (such as types of infections)
Populations at Risk/Individual Risk Factors	Students should gain an understanding of what populations or individuals are most likely to have or to develop a problem with the concept, which is a critical skill for *noticing* as it relates to clinical judgment; help students differentiate populations at risk as opposed to individual risk factors
Physiologic Processes and Consequences	Physiologic processes and consequences typically present the physiologic basis for dysfunction and the consequence (i.e., what the individual experiences)
Assessment • History • Examination findings • Diagnostic tests	At the concept level, this section helps the student identify the individual's status as it relates to the concept (optimal functioning or dysfunction); again, this understanding is critical for clinical judgment
Clinical Management • Primary prevention • Screening • Collaborative interventions	Students must gain a clear understanding of what they should do when encountering the health care recipient as it relates to the concept, which is also a critical element of clinical judgment; this comprehensive look at preventative, screening, or treatment options is performed to enhance or maintain optimal function or treat in situations of dysfunction and is not focused at the disease level but rather at the concept level; when exemplars are taught, the elements within this section should easily connect
Interrelated Concepts	Students should consider how the concept links to other concepts; many concepts have other concepts that are clearly closely interrelated (e.g., perfusion and gas exchange); purposeful learning about these interrelationships establishes the cognitive patterns needed for making future connections
Common Exemplars	Every concept has multiple exemplars; although only a few are formally taught, it is helpful for students to have exposure to applicable exemplars

a balance between faculty-led and student-centered activities. The plan incorporates a situational context for learning enhancement and purposeful linkages to past learning that connects to the students' existing cognitive frameworks, which are critical elements to include in any lesson plan to enhance learning. Also note that the concept presentation does not include a presentation of exemplars, but students are encouraged to consider possible exemplars that link to the concept.

In the sample lesson plan, notice that purposeful connections to other concepts (in all three concept categories) are made. One could make the case that all concepts connect to each other in some way, so the focus should be on the concepts that have the closest connection and greatest impact on the primary concept being discussed. As the interrelated concepts are discussed, the instructor asks the "So what?" question to establish the importance of knowing the typical interrelated concepts for a concept. The present discussion focuses on the commonly

TABLE 6-2 **Concept Presentation Template for Professional Nursing and Health Care Concepts or Health Care Recipient Concepts**

TOPIC	DESCRIPTION
Concept Definitions	A clear definition of the concept should be included so students (and faculty) are all working from a common definition; concept definitions can be easily found in the literature
Scope or Categories of Concept	All concepts have scopes or categories; a scope is like a continuum (such as novice to expert); categories are discrete distinctions (such as leadership styles)
Attributes	Attributes are the critical elements used to correctly identify the concept; they are like the "rule" for acceptance; attributes are essential for clarification related to recognition of the concept in practice
Theoretical Links	Many of the professional nursing concepts and patient attribute concepts have strong links to a theory or theories, such as Tanner's Model of Clinical Judgment; students should gain a perspective about these theories to better understand the concept
Context to Nursing and Health Care	The context to nursing and health care should help the student gain an understanding of the situational context in which the concept will be seen and how it applies to the practice
Interrelated Concepts	Students should consider how the concept links to other concepts; many concepts have other concepts that are clearly closely interrelated (e.g., quality and safety), and purposeful learning about these interrelationships establishes the cognitive patterns needed for making future connections
Common Exemplars	Every concept has multiple exemplars; although only a few are formally taught, it is helpful for students to have exposure to many applicable exemplars

associated interrelated concepts that comprise the enduring understandings about a concept that may apply to every patient. Other interrelated concepts emerge when the concept is applied to a specific clinical context or when specific exemplars are discussed. Another example of a learning activity related to interrelated concepts is presented later in this chapter.

Teaching Exemplars

After the concept presentation, exemplars are taught to give students an opportunity to understand the concept more deeply. An exemplar is an example of a health condition or situation in which the concept under study would be present. It is critical that faculty teach the designated exemplars that best represent the concept (according to the curriculum plan) and to resist the temptation to teach all exemplars from a previous curriculum. Teaching an excessive number of exemplars results in content saturation, with faculty reverting back to intense lectures and students engaging in rote memorization. This outcome minimizes the benefits of the concept-based approach (Giddens & Brady, 2007). Students will have opportunities to learn additional exemplars and to make linkages to concepts during clinical experiences.

TABLE 6-3 Sample Lesson Plan for the Concept of Perfusion

FOCUS AREA	TEACHING STRATEGIES/ACTIVITIES	LEARNING OUTCOME
Concept Introduction	• **Instructor:** Introduces concept definitions, categories (e.g., central perfusion and local perfusion) and scope (e.g., no perfusion, reduced perfusion, and optimal perfusion) • **Learning Groups:** Students share what they have previously learned or seen that links to perfusion categories and/or scopes	Clearly articulates the concept
Concept Identification	• **Instructor:** Presents populations at highest risk for perfusion problems; clarifies how these are similar and different from individual risk factors • **Learning Groups:** Students complete a table identifying common individual risk factors across the life span; groups report and the instructor clarifies answers • **Instructor:** Presents a profile of four persons; students identify individual risk factors for each person • **Instructor:** Makes a presentation focused on how perfusion can become impaired and physiologic consequences with impairment; shows a short video that clearly illustrates this process • **Learning Groups:** Students review assessment skills previously learned in their health assessment class and link data to central perfusion, local perfusion, or both • **Instructor:** Shows photos depicting clinical findings of impaired perfusion; the students describe the relevance of the signs • **Learning Groups:** Students complete a worksheet on common diagnostic tests to evaluate perfusion (central and local)	Recognizes persons with optimal perfusion, those at risk, and those who are experiencing poor perfusion
Clinical Management	• **Learning Groups:** Assign half the groups to locate recommended health promotion strategies from Healthy People 2020 (each group has a different age group) and half the groups to locate recommended screening guidelines from the USPSTF (each group has a different age group); the groups report • **Instructor:** Presents information about clinical treatment guidelines for perfusion problems—procedures, surgical interventions, and pharmacotherapy	Initiates appropriate interventions and assesses patient outcome
Transferable Ideas	• **Learning Groups:** Students will identify up to five curriculum concepts and draw a concept map showing interrelated connections • **Learning Groups:** Students will brainstorm medical conditions they are aware of that represent perfusion problems and identify if it represents a central or peripheral perfusion problem; the instructor will clarify answers and add to lists generated for further consideration	Application of principles to other concepts and clinical conditions
Notes	After the concept overview, the following exemplars will be used to deepen the students' understanding of perfusion: • Heart failure • Acute myocardial infarction • Peripheral vascular disease	

USPSTF, U.S. Preventive Services Task Force.

When faculty teach the exemplar, purposeful linkages back to the concept presentation must be made. Faculty teach exemplars through the use of balanced teaching strategies and within the context of clinical practice. Exemplars provide a link to what students see in practice; they provide a link to content knowledge but with a concept approach to teach care for the patient and all the concepts important to that patient. Exemplars also link to additional interrelated concepts specific to the exemplar. Figure 6-3 demonstrates the relationship among the target concept, interrelated concepts, the exemplar, and other concepts related to the specific exemplar.

Exemplars serve another purpose. Like all nursing knowledge, how concepts apply in practice depends on the situation. Concepts are usually altered and influenced by the context in which they are situated. They are influenced by other concepts relevant to a patient situation. Therefore exemplars presented in the context of a specific patient or practice situation provide a deeper, more meaningful understanding of the concepts and enhance students' skill in knowledge transferability.

Integrated Teaching for a Patient or Situational Context

One of the traits of expert nursing faculty is integrated teaching—that is, framing what is being learned in a situational context (Benner et al., 2010). Situational context helps students understand how the information they are learning is applied in practice, such as with a patient situation or a professional nursing situation. Integrated teaching enhances conceptual learning because it reinforces the purposefulness of the information and facilitates the learners' ability to transfer ideas from one situation to another.

Integrated teaching can be successfully applied in classroom settings in many ways. One of the most commonly used methods is through the use of case studies. Case studies typically focus on a single situation relevant to the topic being studied, although an unfolding case study presents a situation over time. Another alternative is the use of "standardized virtual patients." Standardized virtual patients are fictional characters that support learning throughout a course or curriculum. Students become familiar with each standardized virtual patient (his or her health history, family situation, and living situation, for example), and faculty use these patients on an ongoing basis for a number of learning activities. Several examples of the use of standardized virtual patients have been reported in the nursing literature (Croteau, Howe, Timmons, Nilson, & Parker 2011; Curran, Elfrink, & Mays, 2009; Giddens, 2007; Walsh, 2011). Box 6-2 presents an example of a community of patients. This community of patients is developed by faculty and is unique to the school. Once faculty develop this community of patients, they can share the information with their students using their course management system.

BOX 6-2 **A Community of Patients**

Families Living in Your Community

The Smith Family
White Family
Mom: Debbie, age 38 years, height 5'2", weight 175 lb, works full time, volunteers for her children's activities
Dad: Mike, age 40 years, height 5'10", weight 250 lb, works full time, travels out of town 3 days a week, smokes 2 packs of cigarettes a day, takes medication for depression, recently diagnosed with diabetes mellitus
Son: Michael, age 8 years, easygoing personality, active in sports, good student, asthma for 3 years, frequent urinary tract infections in the winter
Daughter: Julie, age 2 years, attends day care, has frequent ear infections, is stubborn, does well at school but her parents have difficulty controlling her tantrums
Grandfather: Hector, age 75 years, lives in the "Your Community" Nursing Home, has mild dementia, uses a wheelchair after falling and breaking his right hip, has moderate to severe emphysema as a result of smoking but quit smoking 2 years ago

The Garcia Family
Hispanic Family
Mom: Rosa, age 45 years, weight 180 lb, works two jobs, has five children ages 27, 25, 23, 18, and 15 years
Dad: Jesus, age 57 years, weight 230 lb, smokes two packs of cigarettes per day, works as a dry wall installer, states he is able to eat anything, enjoys American food including fried chicken, French fries, fast food, and sweets but continues to eat foods of Mexican culture, visits Mexico every year for 2 weeks
Son: Jose, age 18 years, attends the local community college, smokes cigarettes and occasionally marijuana, volunteers to help neighborhood children learn English
Daughter: Roseanne, age 15 years, had a miscarriage 1 month ago but did not tell her family, earns A's in school, has a steady boyfriend who is occasionally verbally abusive
Relatives and friends of relatives: Every few months, two to three people from Mexico enter as undocumented immigrants and stay with the Garcia family until they can find a permanent place to live.

The Bailey Family
African American Family
Mom: Julie, age 37 years, weight 135 lb, a lawyer, has one child living at home
Dad: Roy: age 45 years, weight 180 lb, has had hypertension for 20 years
Son: Peter, age 15 years, attends a private high school and is a member of the orchestra, plays in a band with friends who smoke marijuana during practices, but Peter refuses to smoke
Grandmother: Lilly, lives at the "Your Community" Nursing Home, has Alzheimer disease, has severe chronic obstructive pulmonary disease from 50 years of smoking but quit smoking because she "just forgot she smoked," has had a heart attack and has chronic heart failure

Developed by Linda Caputi, Inc. 2010. Used with permission.

Link to Preexisting Understanding

As discussed at the beginning of the chapter, faculty can facilitate conceptual learning by providing opportunities for students to construct new knowledge from previous understanding. A teaching strategy that faculty can use to determine students' preexisting understanding about a concept is to engage students in reflective thinking and guided discussion. Students are provided guided questions or a worksheet to complete either as a preclass assignment or an in-class discussion activity. The questions included on the worksheet, of course, depend on the concept and the information you wish the students to recall from prior learning. Box 6-3 provides an example of guided questions used to link to preexisting understanding, specifically related to a concept introduction (as described in Tables 6-1 and 6-2).

This type of classroom activity provides not only an introduction to the concept but also gives students the opportunity to actively engage in thinking about the concept and what it means to them. This activity provides faculty with valuable information about the students' current understanding of the topic and how to direct the classroom discussion. The activity also gives students the opportunity to consider what they already know about the topic and to clarify any misunderstandings they have about the concept. This type of activity sets the stage for a more thorough discussion about the concept.

Another approach that can be used to explore the students' preexisting understanding about the concept is a short questionnaire administered at the beginning of the class (Hardin & Richardson, 2012). Faculty can correct students' misconceptions or acknowledge their understandings as they apply in a nonnursing context while teaching that in a nursing context, the concept may take on a different meaning or be applied differently. Just as the meaning of a word takes on different meanings when used in different contexts, so will the meaning of nursing concepts. For example, the concept of *Family Dynamics*

BOX 6-3 Examples of Discussion Questions for the Concept of Collaboration

1. Based on your readings and/or previous experiences, what does the word "collaborate" mean to you?
2. Describe a situation in which you experienced effective or successful collaboration with others. Why was the collaboration effective or successful?
3. Describe a situation in which you experienced ineffective or unsuccessful collaboration with others. Why was it unsuccessful?

may take on a different meaning for persons apart from the meaning used in a nursing context.

As the student progresses through the nursing program, the meaning of any one concept may expand as it is applied to different populations and settings. It may be difficult for students to shift their ideas about concepts, especially some that are deeply engrained in their belief systems. Concepts related to belief systems can be difficult to unlearn (Hardin & Richardson, 2012). However, identifying and clarifying misconceptions is an important element in helping students to think like a nurse. Active, meaningful learning across the curriculum with multiple exposures to the concept used in nursing is required to guide students to apply the concept from a nursing perspective.

Teaching Strategies for Collaborative, Student-Centered Learning

As mentioned throughout this book, the instructor must abandon teaching practices that emphasize content and facts and adopt student-centered approaches that require active application of information, thus linking learning to concepts within the context of nursing practice.

Although there are multiple teaching strategies that can be used to teach conceptually, there is not a list of teaching strategies exclusively used to teach conceptually. As previously noted, it is the focus on a primary concept with links to interrelated concepts that makes a teaching strategy a concept-based teaching strategy. The learning helps students construct a cognitive framework based on concepts, and thus concepts are the unifying, driving focus of the teaching techniques. Learning activities should actively engage students, focus on a clinical situation, require students to think, and be meaningful. Students should clearly understand how the activity contributes to their learning.

Faculty are often reluctant to have students work in learning groups for fear that students may not participate or lack the expertise to correctly complete the work. The power of collaborative learning is that students engage on a different level than they do when listening to a lecture. When students work in teams, the combined effect of different brains thinking together—particularly if they are encouraged to look for information online or in their textbook—typically results in accurate work. The role of the faculty member, as the facilitator of learning, is to provide guidance as students complete the activities and to redirect if students are arriving at incorrect conclusions. Short collaborative learning activities integrated within faculty-led discussions (as shown in Table 6-3) are very effective for various aspects of the concept or exemplar presentations. This section presents several examples of strategies that can be applied to various aspects of concept or exemplar learning as individual or collaborative learning activities.

Scope/Categories of Concepts

Table 6-4 provides an example of a collaborative in-class learning activity that directs students to discuss the various dimensions of motivation in the context of health care management.

Risk Factor Assessment

Table 6-5 provides an example of a collaborative in-class learning activity for thermoregulation. In this activity, students consider why age groups have different risks for problems associated with thermoregulation. This collaborative work is assigned as an alternative to having an instructor present a slide showing risk factors.

TABLE 6-4 Example of a Teaching Strategy: Scope of Motivation as a Concept

In your learning groups, share examples or situations in health care management you have seen or heard about that illustrate the concept of *Motivation* across the trajectory of no motivation to intrinsic motivation.

LEVEL OF MOTIVATION	EXAMPLE OR SITUATION
Intrinsic *Motivation*	
Extrinsic *Motivation* with self-determination	
Extrinsic *Motivation* without self-determination	
No *Motivation*	

Adapted from TEACH for Nurses for Giddens, J.F. (2013). *Concepts for Nursing Practice.* St. Louis, Mosby.

TABLE 6-5 Example of a Teaching Strategy: Risk Factor Assessment for the Concept of Thermoregulation

Risk Factor Assessment for Thermoregulation

In your learning groups, identify common risk factors for thermoregulation problems across the life span.

INFANTS AND CHILDREN	ADOLESCENTS AND YOUNG ADULTS	OLDER ADULTS	CONCLUSIONS: HOW ARE RISK FACTORS SIMILAR? HOW ARE THEY DIFFERENT?

Adapted from TEACH for Nurses for Giddens, J.F. (2013). *Concepts for Nursing Practice.* St. Louis, Mosby.

Interventions for Health Promotion

Box 6-4 shows an example of a collaborative learning activity for the concept of *Health Promotion* that focuses on interventions. Student groups prepare posters for an in-class poster health fair outlining the current evidence for health promotion and health screening for various topics. Students learn from each other about the topics rather than from a faculty-driven presentation.

Interrelated Concepts

Students also complete in-class learning activities focusing on interrelated concepts. Identification of the closest interrelated concepts often provides clues to other areas requiring consideration and assessment (Box 6-5).

Concept Exemplars

Table 6-6 presents an example of a collaborative in-class learning activity in which students access the website of the Centers for Disease Control and Prevention

---

BOX 6-4 An Example of a Collaborative Learning Activity for Health Promotion

Interventions for Health Promotion

In your learning groups you will create a poster highlighting current evidence-based recommendations for your assigned health promotion topic. Be sure to include the parameters of the guidelines, particularly for specified population groups or persons with known risk factors, as appropriate. Include your reference. After groups have developed their posters, a poster fair will be held, and each group will share with others the key points for their topics.

BOX 6-5 An Example of a Collaborative Learning Activity for Interrelated Concepts

Interrelated Concepts: Development

Consider the following concepts previously learned in your courses:
- *Culture*
- *Family Dynamics*
- *Genetics*
- *Nutrition*
- *Sensory Perception*

In your learning groups, discuss the relationship of these concepts to the concept of *Development*. Draw a concept map showing the relationships.

TABLE 6-6 **Example of a Teaching Strategy: Identifying Common Exemplars for the Concept of Infection by Age Group**

Common Exemplars of Infection

In your learning groups, visit the website of the Centers for Disease Control and Prevention and identify the 10 most common reported infections by age group.

INFANTS AND CHILDREN	ADOLESCENTS AND YOUNG ADULTS	OLDER ADULTS	CONCLUSIONS: HOW ARE THESE SIMILAR AND DIFFERENT?

Adapted from TEACH for Nurses for Giddens, J.F. (2013). *Concepts for Nursing Practice.* St. Louis, Mosby.

---

to determine the most common types of infections in the United States (or their state) by age group. This activity links to the concept presentation and helps students gain an awareness of the broad range of exemplars they are likely to encounter in clinical practice. It is again important to reinforce the fact that instructors will not be teaching all the exemplars listed.

Concept Maps

Student-developed concept maps provide a window into the mind of the student as he or she diagrams how concepts interrelate (Caputi & Blach, 2008). Students work in pairs or small groups to first develop simple maps and then expand those maps to demonstrate a growing complexity of concepts throughout the curriculum. For example, students work individually or in small groups to develop a concept map showing the relationship between anxiety and other concepts. Students then discuss their rationale for the relationships made.

Compare and Contrast

An excellent teaching strategy to promote thinking is comparing and contrasting similar situations or opposite ends of a spectrum. This technique can be used as an in-class collaborative learning activity or students can complete it independently, after which the results can be used as discussion points in class. Table 6-7 provides an example of comparing and contrasting suppressed and exaggerated immune responses. The compare and contrast technique can be used for a number of different concepts in many different ways.

TABLE 6-7 **Example of a Teaching Strategy: Compare and Contrast Degrees of Immunity**	
As a group activity, students create a list of common symptoms and clinical findings associated with suppressed and exaggerated immunity and then discuss why each symptom or clinical finding occurs from a physiologic perspective.	
SUPPRESSED IMMUNITY: COMMON CLINICAL FINDINGS	**EXAGGERATED IMMUNITY: COMMON CLINICAL FINDINGS**

Adapted from TEACH for Nurses for Giddens, J.F. (2013). *Concepts for Nursing Practice*. St. Louis, Mosby.

Questions That Promote Thinking

Faculty can challenge students to apply their thinking by presenting questions in the classroom for students to answer. Typically this activity is performed using an audience response system. Once students have considered the question, before providing the answer, ask students to discuss their answers with a fellow student who answered differently. The students should discuss their answers and the rationales for their answers. They will either convince their peer to change his or her answer or change their own answer based on new insights. Students engage in deep, meaningful learning as they are discussing their thinking processes with their peers. Of course, to be a conceptual learning method, the questions must be focused on concepts and not bits of information about the topic (Hardin & Richardson, 2012).

Developing Enduring Understandings and Thinking Skills

A primary purpose of active learning strategies that focus on concepts is to build enduring understandings—that is, discovering the concepts that interrelate and their enduring relationships across populations, diseases, and environments.

Students must be taught to think so they can develop enduring understandings. The active learning strategies described in this chapter guide students through the thinking process. By engaging in these activities, they are not just learning information but are gaining insight into the way a nurse thinks. Guided thinking activities in the context of the concepts help students develop their metacognitive skills, or the ability to understand and monitor their thinking. Metacognition is a critical skill for nurses to practice. The goal of developing metacognition is achieved by making the learning process explicit with regard to learning how to think. The volume of information nurses must process each day requires learning how to approach thinking so the information becomes meaningful and endures across patient populations.

Applying Concept-Based Teaching in Clinical Experiences

The current model for clinical education needs to be addressed for many reasons. Ironside and McNelis (2010) conducted a research study on clinical learning that was very revealing. Based on this study, the authors report that students reported the following outcomes with regard to their clinical education:

1. They had too much "down time"
2. Too much time was focused on performing repetitive tasks that do not result in new learning
3. Too little time was focused on learning higher order thinking skills

It is likely that many clinical hours fail to result in productive learning. Students spend much of their clinical time performing routine care tasks repeatedly, which may not contribute significantly to increased learning. Faculty report spending most of their time supervising students in hands-on procedures, leaving little time to focus on fostering the development of clinical reasoning skills (Institute of Medicine [IOM], 2010; Ironside & McNelis, 2010).

Toward a New Clinical Model

The old clinical model of providing total patient care as the primary clinical activity, which has been the model for more than 50 years, is no longer working as a means for students to learn to provide safe, quality nursing care (IOM, 2010; Tanner, 2010). According to Tanner, the following foci for learning activities, along with others, can better prepare students for safe practice:

- Deepening and extending theoretical knowledge and learning how key concepts are exemplified in practice
- Developing skill in clinical judgment and other thinking skills and strategies; clinical judgment requires guided practice in working through patient situations in a number of different contexts as they unfold in the clinical setting
- Developing an understanding of the culture of health care and nursing and how the health care system functions, especially as it relates to the patient, the role of the nurse, and interaction with other interprofessional health care providers

These foci can be addressed in a concept-based curriculum.

A change in the approach to teaching clinical skills may appear to be impossible, but it can and has changed for many faculty at all levels of nursing education, especially in prelicensure programs. A focus on concepts provides a basis for making this necessary change. The three foci presented by Tanner (2010) can be used to design clinical activities based on a concept-based curriculum approach as shown in the following discussion.

Extending Theoretical Knowledge

Tanner's first focus is deepening and extending theoretical knowledge and learning how key concepts are exemplified in practice (Tanner, 2010). After a concept is introduced in class, students in the clinical experience focus on that concept. For example, the concept of *Safety* is introduced in a beginning nursing course. During the clinical experience, two students will not be assigned traditional patient care but will complete an assignment focused on the concept of *Safety*. The assignment presented in Box 6-6 is used for this activity.

The students who complete this activity discuss the results in postconference. The other students also discuss how the National Patient Safety Goals were or were not evident in the care of their patients. Additionally, other safety measures related to their assigned patients are discussed. The following clinical day, two different students may focus on the concept of *Health Care Quality*, demonstrating how that concept relates to the concept of *Safety*.

BOX 6-6 Active Learning Activity for the Concept of Safety

National Patient Safety Goals

Two students print the National Patient Safety Goals for the environment in which they are working. These two students spend one day assessing the environment and at least three patients. Their goal is to look at the environment and these patients from the perspective of the Joint Commission's National Patient Safety Goals. The students address the following questions.

Questions

1. What precautions should the nurse take with regard to each safety goal for each patient?
2. For each patient, is one particular safety goal the most important?
3. What information about each of these patients is most important to communicate to the nurse on the next shift?
4. What factors regarding the environment indicate that these safety goals are being met?
    Gap analysis: What factors regarding the environment indicate a need for change so the safety goals can be met?

Developing Clinical Judgment

The second focus presented by Tanner (2010) addresses the development of clinical judgment and other thinking skills and strategies. According to Nielsen and Lasater (2013), the concept of *Clinical Judgment* generally refers to *"interpretations and inferences that influence actions in clinical practice"* (p. 365). Simply providing students with this, or another, definition of clinical judgment and then asking them to apply clinical judgment to their care is not very helpful and does not ensure that the student can apply clinical judgment when needed.

Clinical Judgment is a concept that needs to be taught beginning in the first nursing course. Clinical judgment requires guided practice in working through patient situations in a number of different contexts as they unfold in the clinical setting. Guided instruction in clinical judgment is critical for students to learn to think like a nurse. When they enter the nursing program, students are at the novice level. They are not familiar with the nursing profession and have no knowledge of how nurses solve problems. How might a faculty member in the clinical setting provide guided instruction for students to engage in clinical judgment? Before a nurse can use interpretations and inferences to influence actions, information must be collected, but what information should be collected? Novice students need specific guidance to learn to think like a nurse.

When engaging in clinical judgment, nurses must make decisions based on data, but they first must know what information to collect, then interpret the meaning of the data, and finally act on that data. This type of thinking can be taught in the first nursing course when students are learning about vital signs. Students learn the normal ranges for vital signs. Novice learners use these norms as the rule used to determine if the patient's vital signs are acceptable. They do not yet know that, depending on the context, readings outside the normal range may be acceptable. The activity in Box 6-7 provides guided practice in applying the concept of *Clinical Judgment* as students collect the data that a nurse uses to determine if a patient's vital signs are acceptable.

This activity guides the students through a basic application of the concept of *Clinical Judgment* and helps teach the students how to think like a nurse. All students are learning that normal values are only guidelines. Actual patient data may be outside the normal range, but by collecting the appropriate data and then making *interpretations and inferences* about the data, conclusions are made that guide *actions in clinical practice*. This activity brings to life that definition of clinical judgment. The significance of the vital signs is determined within the context of each of the individual patients. This activity helps move students past the novice stage of clinical expertise, at which point they want to apply all rules to all patients.

> ### BOX 6-7 Example of a Clinical Activity for the Concept of Clinical Judgment
>
> 1. Two students take vital signs for three patients and collect the following information for each of the three patients: age, range of vital sign readings for the past 24 hours, medications the patient is currently taking, information about the medications that may affect the vital signs, disease/condition that brought the patient to the health care setting, information about the disease/condition that may influence vital signs, other preexisting conditions and their effect on the vital signs, any procedures the patient experienced while in the health care setting and the effect of those procedures on vital signs, and activity level.
> 2. During the postconference, the two students present the first patient and the patient's current vital signs and then discuss each of the additional pieces of information. The faculty may assist with explanations about information the students have not yet learned, such as pathophysiology.
> 3. After presenting all the information, the students make decisions about the vital signs:
>   - Are they acceptable, even if they are not in the normal range? Why? Why not?
>   - How high or how low can each of the patient's vital signs vary without causing alarm?
>   - If the patient's vital signs are outside that range, does additional information need to be collected, and who will you notify?
> 4. The second patient is presented. The same information is addressed. Upon completion of the discussion about the second patient, comparisons are made between the first patient and the second patient, with a discussion about why the vital signs for each patient vary.
> 5. The third patient is presented and is also compared with the first two patients.

© 2013, Linda Caputi, Inc. Used with permission.

The activity helps students appreciate that rules are guidelines that only have meaning within the context of a particular patient.

This lesson in the way nurses think is then applied by students when making decisions about other patient data. The students may not always know what data to collect, but they have learned that clinical judgment requires collecting and interpreting data, and thus appropriate data must first be collected. As they advance through the program and broaden their knowledge base, they become more skilled at identifying the specific data they should collect.

This activity is just one example of how a faculty member can guide students' thinking as they apply the concept of *Clinical Judgment*. These types of activities should be numerous and varied throughout every clinical course. Nurses use a variety of thinking skills and strategies as they engage in clinical judgment, and students should be guided through the process of applying each of these skills and strategies in the clinical setting. Appendix A provides additional tools to use in the clinical setting.

Culture of Health Care

The third focus suggested by Tanner (2010) relates to the culture of health care and nursing and how the health care system functions. The traditional model for clinical instruction places the students in the patients' rooms for the majority of the time they are in the clinical setting. It is important for students to engage in direct patient care. However, time must also be spent learning about the health care environment. Spector and Echternacht (2011) report that a number of studies have cited actual errors and near misses that have resulted from a lack of familiarity with the workplace environment. Students must learn about the culture of health care and can do so by studying the concept of *Health Care Organizations* while in the clinical setting. Box 6-8 presents an example of the application of the concept of *Health Care Organizations* in the clinical setting.

The importance of safe administration of medications cannot be overemphasized. However, many faculty focus exclusively on the actual psychomotor skill of administering the medication. Although this aspect of medication administration is extremely important, students might engage in many other activities that relate to the functioning of the health care system and represent important learning for the purpose of safe administration of medications. Focusing on the entire process of medication administration within the framework of the concept of *Health Care Organization* is critical not only to avoid errors in medication administration but to identify potential problems and work to resolve them before an error is made.

Box 6-8 **The Concept of Health Care Organizations**

Medication Administration from a Systems Perspective

- Two students work with two different nurses on day 1 and then two different nurses on day 2 (four nurses total). (If this is a 12-hour clinical day, the student works with one nurse for ½ of the shift then a different nurse for the other ½ of the shift to simulate two 6 hour days.) The students should "shadow" each nurse, watching and noting *every* step of the system pertaining to the administration of medications—from the time the medication order is written until the effects of that medication have been evaluated.
- Halfway through the second day of the experience, the two students work together to develop a description of the system used in that health care agency. They might develop a chart, a concept map, or any other visualization of the process.
- The students then describe and discuss the health care system in the postconference. They focus on the elements of the larger system and where in the process an error might be made— and by whom—that can result in a medication error by the nurse.
- The students then compare and contrast the current system with the medication system in another type of health care institution. How are they the same? How are they different?

Additional Teaching Strategies for the Clinical Setting

Psychomotor Skills

Concept-based teaching strategies related to psychomotor skills can be used in the clinical setting. For example, two students may be assigned to assess three different patients chosen by faculty to determine how to safely alter selected skills procedures learned in the nursing skills laboratory. The faculty selects three skills for the activity. The students engage in the following activity:

1. Review the procedure learned for three psychomotor skills: inserting a urinary catheter, starting an intravenous line, and changing a complicated abdominal dressing.
2. The two students assess each of the three patients.
3. The students work together to determine how each of the three nursing skills will be modified for each of the three patients assessed.
4. The modifications will then be explained in terms of concepts. For example, if a patient cannot lay flat because of gas exchange issues, positioning for insertion of a urinary catheter would be modified. The student would identify gas exchange as the concept addressed with the modification.

Patient Assessment

Another clinical activity involves the assessment of patients by students. Students must learn to assess a patient and be able to identify patient needs that have not been identified through a shift or Situation-Background-Assessment-Recommendation report. Each student in the clinical group enters a different patient's room without any knowledge of the patient or the patient's condition. Each student performs an assessment of his or her assigned patient. The students then leave the room and list everything they observed. They determine what concepts their assessment data represent. They then identify interrelated concepts for each of the identified concepts. From their list of concepts, they develop a list of nursing actions (such as gather more data from laboratory reports and review the medication administration record) and nursing interventions to address the identified concepts. Finally, they prioritize the nursing interventions and explain their decisions. Please note that students will not perform patient care. They are performing an assessment before leaving the room to complete the rest of the assignment.

Clinical Activity Related to a Concept Introduced in Theory

It is important to relate theory to clinical practice. For example, during the week that the concept of *Infection* is introduced in the classroom, the clinical experience focuses on infection. Table 6-8 presents a focused assignment for two students in the clinical

TABLE 6-8 **Example of a Teaching Strategy: Compare and Contrast Patients with an Infection**

Compare and Contrast Three Patients with an Infection

FACTORS TO CONSIDER	PATIENT 1	PATIENT 2	PATIENT 3
Type of infection/pathophysiology			
Preexisting conditions			
Medications prescribed			
Age-related considerations			
Attributes of the concept of *Infection* most affecting the patient			
Interrelated concepts			
CONCEPTS TO CONSIDER	**PATIENT 1**	**PATIENT 2**	**PATIENT 3**
Care Coordination			
Patient Education			
Developmental Level			
Health Care Environment			
Health Promotion			
Ethics			
Add other concepts important to these patients			

group. The two students study the three patients and complete the table. Other students are assigned to provide nursing care to these patients.

During postconference, the two students present the information they gathered. All students engage in the discussion, comparing and contrasting the three patients. As noted, the central focus of the discussion is the concept of *Infection*.

As these examples demonstrate, a concept-based curriculum can be implemented in the clinical setting in many ways. Many activities can be used to engage students in meaningful learning. Faculty must deliberately plan new activities in the clinical setting to ensure students are engaged in learning that is focused on concepts rather than primarily on diseases and alterations of various body systems.

Summary

As evidenced by the variety of teaching strategies presented in this chapter, many teaching methods are used in a concept-based curriculum. Only a sampling of activities were presented. The primary guideline is that learning activities be deliberately planned, with concepts being the major organizing factor. The second Misconceptions and Clarifications Box presents one last misconception in this chapter on teaching/learning strategies for the concept-based curriculum.

Misconceptions and Clarifications

Misconception: Once a concept-based curriculum is in place, all faculty will teach the curriculum in the way it was intended.

Clarification: Many faculty are comfortable teaching in the traditional style and in a very linear fashion. Additionally, many students are comfortable with the traditional approach and may be resistant to concept-based, active learning strategies. These two factors often result in faculty teaching in the same manner as they always have rather than with a concept-based approach. Unfortunately, this scenario results in a concept-based curriculum on paper but not in action. Therefore, evaluation data about the effectiveness of the concept-based curriculum are not reflective of a concept-based curriculum but of a traditional curriculum. It is important for faculty to teach the concept-based curriculum in the way it was intended so evaluation data can accurately reflect the intent and effects of the curriculum.

REFERENCES

Benner P, Sutphen M, Leonard V, Day L: *Educating nurses: A call for radical transformation*, San Francisco, CA, 2010, Jossey-Bass.

Benner P, Tanner C, Chesla C: In *Expertise in nursing practice: Caring, clinical judgment, and ethics*, 2nd ed., New York, NY, 2009, Springer.

Caputi L: An overview of the educational process. In Caputi L, editor: *Teaching nursing the art and science*, 2nd ed., vol. 1. Glen Ellyn, IL, 2010a, DuPage Press, pp 27–47.

Caputi L: An introduction to developing critical thinking in nursing students. In Caputi L, editor: *Teaching nursing the art and science*, 2nd ed., vol. 2. Glen Ellyn, IL, 2010b, DuPage Press, pp 381–390.

Caputi L, Blach D: *Teaching nursing using concept maps*, Glen Ellyn, IL, 2008, DuPage Press.

Croteau SD, Howe LA, Timmons SM, Nilson L, Parker VG: Evaluation of the effectiveness of "The Village": A pharmacology education teaching strategy, *Nursing Education Perspectives* 32(5):338–341, 2011.

Curran R, Elfrink V, Mays B: Building a virtual community for nursing education: The town of Mirror Lake, *Journal of Nursing Education* 48(1):30–35, 2009.

Giddens JF: The Neighborhood: A web-based platform to support conceptual teaching and learning, *Nursing Education Perspectives* 28(5):251–256, 2007.

Giddens JF, Brady DP: Rescuing nursing education from content saturation: The case for a concept-based curriculum, *Journal of Nursing Education* 46(2):65–69, 2007.

Hardin PK, Richardson SJ: Teaching the concept curricula: Theory and method, *Journal of Nursing Education* 51(3):155–159, 2012.

Institute of Medicine: *A summary of the February 2010 forum on the future of nursing*, Washington, DC, 2010, The National Academies Press.

Ironside P, McNelis A: *Clinical education in prelicensure nursing programs: Results from an NLN national survey*, New York, NY, 2010, National League for Nursing.

Nielsen A, Lasater K: In Giddens JF, editor: *Concepts for nursing practice*, St. Louis, MO, 2013, Mosby Elsevier.

Schunk DH: *Learning theories: An educational perspective*, 6th ed., Upper Saddle River, NJ, 2012, Pearson.

Spector N, Echternacht M: A regulatory model for transitioning newly licensed nurses to practice, *Journal of Nursing Regulation* 1(2):18–25, 2011.

Tanner C: From mother duck to mother lode: Clinical education for deep learning, *Journal of Nursing Education* 49(1):3–4, 2010.

Walsh M: Narrative pedagogy and simulation: Future directions for nursing education, *Nurse Education in Practice* 11:216–219, 2011.

Evaluation of Student Learning

7

Linda Caputi

Evaluation of student learning is a fundamental component of education. However, because learning occurs in the mind and thus cannot be directly measured or observed, student learning is difficult to measure. In the 1950s, a common behavioral theory definition of learning was that it results in a *change* in behavior, and thus we can really only infer that learning has occurred on the basis of observed behavior. Although the idea of *change* permeates most definitions of learning, the definition of learning has expanded since the early behavioral theory–based studies as a result of the influence of newer learning theories. Because this book focuses on the cognitive processing of students while they are involved in learning, a definition that includes the notion of change but also captures the higher-level cognitive processing of students is more functional. One such definition of learning is, "Learning is a process that brings together cognitive, emotional, and environmental influences and experiences for acquiring, enhancing, or making changes in one's knowledge, skills, values, and worldviews" (Merriam, Caffarella, & Baumgartner, 2007, p. 277). This definition aligns nicely with the concept-based teaching strategies discussed in Chapter 6. This definition also demonstrates that evaluation of learning is complex and requires a variety of assessment methods.

Evaluation of student learning is an important component of the conceptual approach, and this evaluation is performed at both the individual student level and the program level. Evaluation methods must ensure assessment of learning outcomes as they relate to the program's framework, which is based on concepts. This chapter expands on the information presented in Chapter 4 regarding program evaluation and presents best practices to evaluate student learning at both the course level and the program level to determine the effectiveness of a concept-based curriculum.

Program Evaluation Plan

As mentioned in Chapter 4, a program evaluation plan is designed as part of curriculum development. An evaluation plan is a critical component in determining the effectiveness of a new concept-based curriculum. The evaluation plan should be a proactive and systematic process that is developed to determine if the curriculum is achieving the desired outcomes (Davis, Grinnell, & Niemer, 2013). Nursing faculty are familiar with curriculum evaluation plans as a key requirement for accreditation. These plans—which include assessment of curricular outcomes, frequency of assessments for which data are collected, analysis of the data, interpretation of the findings, and plans for using the data to guide program improvement (Accreditation Commission for Education in Nursing [ACEN], 2013a; Commission on Collegiate Nursing Education [CCNE], 2014)—can be applied to evaluating the effectiveness of a concept-based curriculum. If the data indicate that any of the outcomes are not being met, faculty should use these data to guide program changes.

Learning Outcomes

Learning outcomes are "Statements of expectations written in measurable terms that express what a student will know, do, or think at the end of a learning experience; characteristics of the student at the completion of a course and/or program. Learning outcomes are measurable, learner-oriented abilities that are consistent with standards of professional practice" (ACEN, 2013b, p. 5). *Program learning outcomes* reflect the characteristics or attributes of the students at the end of the nursing program. These learning outcomes represent the types of behaviors and activities students are able to engage in by the end of the curriculum. In the past, program learning outcomes were called "terminal objectives," an old term that is no longer used in nursing education with an outcomes-based curriculum. *Course learning outcomes* reflect the characteristics or attributes of the students at the end of a nursing course.

Program learning outcomes are carefully developed by faculty to reflect institutional educational expectations and national standards. Once established, the program learning outcomes are used to develop the course learning outcomes. The course learning outcomes are then used to develop the course outlines and lesson objectives for each classroom session. A course calendar is developed that focuses on the concepts and exemplars, as well as teaching methods for each class session. Evaluation methods align with the expectations of the course. Use of a variety of methods to evaluate learning and program outcomes is not new to a concept-based curriculum. All these components provide a sound, internally consistent curriculum. Figure 7-1 demonstrates this flow.

The final step in the process illustrated in Figure 7-1 is evaluation. Many assessment methods are used to evaluate student achievement of lesson objectives that—because all curricular components are linked—are a measurement of course

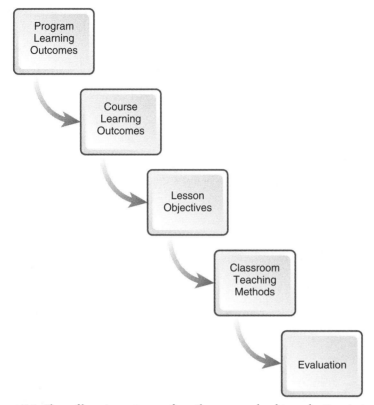

Figure 7-1 Flow of learning outcomes from the program level to evaluation strategies.

learning outcomes. Student learning in a concept-based curriculum is assessed with use of the same evaluation processes that are part of any nursing curriculum. The primary difference for the concept-based curriculum is that the evaluation methods must ensure assessment of learning outcomes as they relate to the program's framework, which is based on concepts. These evaluation methods are varied and include examinations, clinical evaluation tools, formal papers, student presentations, student surveys, and faculty surveys. As students successfully complete each course in the nursing program, the course learning outcomes build to culminate in the program learning outcomes. Achievement of the program learning outcomes should then result in positive program outcomes.

Program Outcomes

Program outcomes represent a different set of outcomes than the *program learning outcomes.* Program outcomes are "Indicators that reflect the extent to which the purposes of the nursing education unit are achieved and by which program effectiveness is documented. Program outcomes are measurable, consumer-oriented indexes designed to evaluate the degree to which the program is achieving its mission and goals. Examples include but are not limited to: program completion rates, job placement rates, licensure/certification exam pass rates, graduate satisfaction, and employer satisfaction" (ACEN, 2013b, p. 4). If a nursing program curriculum is well planned and deliberately delivered, the program outcomes should be achieved through achievement of the program learning outcomes.

Evaluating Learning Outcomes

 Misconceptions and Clarifications

Misconception: The conceptual approach requires completely different strategies to evaluate student learning.	**Clarification:** Faculty will continue to use many of the same evaluation strategies, but with a different focus. The focus of evaluation for the conceptual approach is the students' ability to transfer information from one situation to another. A focus on the application of conceptual understanding is at the heart of evaluation of student learning.

It is the responsibility of the nursing faculty to determine if students have achieved the program learning outcomes by measuring achievement of course learning outcomes through the application of valid and reliable evaluation methods. These evaluation methods are varied and include examinations, clinical evaluation tools, formal papers, classroom presentations, and portfolios, among others. The key to measuring learning outcomes is that each evaluation tool should demonstrate a connection to a learning outcome that relates to the concept-based curriculum. Student performance should be clearly linked to the application of the concept used in the curriculum. Consider the following example from an Advanced Adult Health course:

Program Learning Outcome

- Participate in collaboration and teamwork with members of the interprofessional team, the patient, and the patient's support persons. The concepts addressed include *Collaboration* and *Communication.*

Course Learning Outcome

- Compare and contrast techniques used to develop collaborative relationships with members of the interprofessional team, the patient, and the patient's support persons when caring for patients with complex, high-acuity conditions.

Lesson Objective

- The faculty developing a lesson plan to teach to this learning outcome may then develop *a lesson objective,* such as: Analyze inter- and intraprofessional communication and collaborative skills used to deliver safe, evidence-based, patient-centered care.

Classroom Teaching Methods

- Teaching strategies are planned that engage students in learning about collaboration at the analysis level.

Evaluation

- Evaluation methods to measure this course learning outcome are then developed. A variety of methods such as classroom examinations, projects, and the clinical evaluation tool are used.

A critical part of evaluating student learning in any curriculum, but especially in the concept-based curriculum, is transfer of learning. Faculty evaluate students' ability to transfer learning about a concept from one situation to another to answer the question, *Can the students use what they have learned in a new situation?* All learning should be transferable to new situations. Just as a child who learns multiplication tables must be able to determine when to use that math skill, so it is with the learning of concepts. Students who learn about a concept must be able to discern when knowledge of that concept should be used in a particular context. Evaluation methods provide opportunities for students to demonstrate that they are able to apply their learning to new situations.

Classroom Examinations

One method for evaluating student achievement of course learning outcomes is a classroom examination. The faculty use a test blueprint that directly links a test item to the lesson objective, which is linked to the course learning outcome. If students are able to answer the test items linked to the lesson objective and the test items are determined to be reliable on the basis of item analysis, faculty can determine that students are achieving the course learning outcome related to a given concept.

Classroom examinations cover concepts taught during the classroom sessions, as well as the exemplars used for concept application. For example, with regard to the *lesson objective* example in the previous section, a test item focused on the concept of *Collaboration* may have the following stem:

Present a patient situation. Then ask: ***Which collaborative action will the nurse take?***

This question is focused on a patient situation while asking a question about the concept of *Collaboration*. An alternate approach to evaluating students' understanding of *Collaboration* is to present a question that asks the student what action the nurse will take. The actions listed in the options reflect a number of different concepts, of which one represents a *Collaboration* behavior without using the word "collaboration." The correct answer is the option representing *Collaboration*. This type of question evaluates the students' understanding of when to apply *Collaboration* to a situation rather than an action representing another concept.

The cognitive level of questions should match the course learning outcomes. The questions should assess the understanding of concepts via application and analysis of the concepts at a level appropriate to the course. For example, a simple application question may be:

Present a patient situation. ***Which concepts will the nurse further investigate?***

The stem of this question does not ask about a specific concept; rather, students must draw from the patient situation the concepts that will be further investigated.

Questions directed at the application of concepts related to exemplars are also included on examinations. An example of a question related to the concept of *Pain* experienced by a patient during the postoperative period may be:

The nurse assesses a patient 2 days after abdominal surgery. The patient reports diffuse abdominal discomfort. The nurse notes few bowel sounds, distention, and lack of flatus. ***The nurse should implement which intervention?***

All the aforementioned questions represent a focus on concepts applied to patient situations. By using a test blueprint to link each question to a course learning outcome that represents specific concepts, the faculty can analyze test results to determine which questions did and did not result in good student performance. This analysis provides information about student achievement of specific learning outcomes and the concepts related to those learning outcomes. This information is necessary to guide the faculty's actions to improve the course on the basis of poor performance related to identified learning outcomes.

Clinical Evaluation Tools

Clinical evaluation tools are commonly used to assess student performance. These tools are used to measure achievement of course learning outcomes as they relate to the clinical environment. Again, if the course learning outcomes represent important nursing concepts, then evaluation of the course learning outcomes in turn evaluates student learning with regard to the application of the concepts used to build the curriculum.

Continuing with the example of *Collaboration*, an item on the clinical evaluation tool is developed to evaluate this concept. The course learning outcome presented earlier can be used for this purpose: *Compare and contrast techniques used to develop collaborative relationships with members of the interprofessional team, the patient, and the patient's support persons when caring for patients with complex, high-acuity conditions.*

Students then engage in clinical activities that demonstrate their ability to analyze *Collaboration*. Box 7-1 presents a clinical learning activity that can be used for this purpose. This activity is a focused exercise that directs the students to observe the activities and behaviors of the interprofessional team for the purpose of learning to deal with conflict, an important communication skill used when engaging in a collaborative relationship. The activity is best graded with use of a grading rubric. The use of a rubric ensures a more objective evaluation by faculty, as well as consistent grading among faculty with different groups of students. Table 7-1 presents a grading rubric.

BOX 7-1 Sample Clinical Learning Activity for Conflict Resolution

1. Interview a nurse and one other health care professional to identify an area of conflict in the clinical area.
   - Nurse:
   - Health Care Professional:
2. Ask the nurse and health care professional how the conflict was resolved.
   - Nurse:
   - Health Care Professional:
3. Observe the interactions of all the health care professionals on the unit. What conflicts did you observe? How were they handled or not handled?
4. Using conflict resolution principles, how would you approach this conflict?

   Explain your approach.

TABLE 7-1 Grading Rubric for Conflict Resolution Clinical Activity

PERFORMANCE CRITERIA	SATISFACTORY	NEEDS IMPROVEMENT	UNSATISFACTORY
Conflicts identified on the unit	Clearly describes conflicts on the unit	Descriptions of conflicts on the unit are vague and unclear	Unable to describe any conflicts on the unit
Explanation of how to resolve a conflict	Clearly and accurately explains how to handle the conflict	Explanation of handling the conflict is scant and not well substantiated	Unable to explain how to handle the conflict

This conflict resolution activity is used to evaluate individual student performance related to the identified course learning outcome. However, the activity can also be used to evaluate the class on their performance as a group. Faculty aggregate the scores of all students completing the assignment. The aggregate score is then used to determine if the class as a group is performing well on the assignment. For example, important evaluation information is the percentage of students who completed this assignment with a satisfactory score, as well as the percentage who completed each item on the grading rubric with a satisfactory score. This aggregate score provides information about the level of learning for the class, indicating areas of strength and weaknesses of the course and the curriculum. Any indication of poor performance prompts faculty to determine changes that might be made to enhance the students' learning of the concept of *Collaboration*.

Written Assignments

Written assignments are an important evaluation method. Formal papers provide opportunities for students to demonstrate not only their knowledge of a concept but their ability to apply higher-level thinking.

Once again using the concept of *Collaboration*, a writing assignment is developed. The course learning outcome presented earlier can be used for this purpose: *Compare and contrast techniques used to develop collaborative relationships with members of the interprofessional team, the patient, and the patient's support persons when caring for patients with complex, high-acuity conditions.* This assignment is for a course at the upper level because it requires students to have had clinical experiences in several different agencies. The purpose of the paper is for the student to compare and contrast collaboration among the interprofessional team members in two health care settings. The assignment is presented in Box 7-2, and a general grading rubric for the assignment is presented in Table 7-2.

Concept Maps to Evaluate Conceptual Linkages

Concept maps are a helpful formative evaluation tool. A concept map is a visual tool that requires the student to organize information and make connections (Caputi & Blach, 2008). As students start their day in the clinical setting, they begin to build a concept map, with the patient in the center of the map. As the student works through the day—performing assessments, making decisions, deciding on interventions, and engaging in the work of a nurse—the student adds to the concept map. The entries on the concept map represent concepts. The student demonstrates links between and among the concepts. Faculty provide immediate feedback as the student builds the concept map throughout the day. This tool

---

BOX 7-2 **Sample Paper Guidelines for the Concept of Collaboration**

Goal of Assignment: Compare and contrast *Collaboration* among members of the health care team in two health care settings.
1. Using the following three attributes of the concept of *Collaboration*, discuss how collaboration among the members of the health care team in each of the settings was similar and how it was different.
   - Roles and responsibilities
   - Communication
   - Teams and teamwork
2. For the concept of *Collaboration*, choose two interrelated concepts. Discuss how they were exemplified in each of the settings. Discuss how the settings were the same and different.
3. Draw conclusions about the collaboration you experienced in each of the health care settings. Discuss and explain why you would choose one setting over the other. Provide rationales for your selection.

TABLE 7-2 **A Sample Grading Rubric**

GRADING RUBRIC	EXCELLENT: 3 POINTS	GOOD: 2 POINTS	FAIR: 1 POINT	UNACCEPTABLE: 0 POINTS
1. Using the following three attributes of the concept of *Collaboration*, discuss how collaboration among the members of the health care team in each of the settings was similar and how it was different	Discussion is complete, explicit, and focused	Discussion is complete and clearly written with minor areas incomplete	Discussion is generally complete but lacks significant information	Discussion is scant, superficial, and lacking in detail
2. For the concept of *Collaboration*, choose two interrelated concepts, discuss how they were exemplified in each of the settings, and discuss how the settings were the same and different	Discussion is complete, explicit, and focused	Discussion is complete and clearly written with minor areas incomplete	Discussion is generally complete but lacks significant information	Discussion is scant, superficial, and lacking in detail
3. Draw conclusions about the collaboration you experienced in each of the health care settings; discuss and explain why you would choose on setting over the other, providing rationales for your selection	Discussion is complete, explicit, and focused	Discussion is complete and clearly written with minor areas incomplete	Discussion is generally complete but lacks significant information	Discussion is scant, superficial, and lacking in detail

provides faculty with a wealth of knowledge about the students' understanding of concepts and linkages among interrelated concepts.

These evaluation methods are examples of measurements of learning outcomes. In a concept-based curriculum, it is important that the evaluation methods used to evaluate student achievement of learning outcomes be linked to concepts so the evaluation of concepts is clearly delineated.

Program Evaluation

Program evaluation looks at achievement of learning outcomes and program outcomes.

Measuring Student Perception of Achievement of Course Learning Outcomes

Feedback from students about the effectiveness of courses in helping them achieve the course learning outcomes is imperative for ongoing program improvement. The completion of course evaluations by students is a well-established practice in education and should be used in the concept-based curriculum. Course evaluations completed by students are focused on the course learning outcomes. All course learning outcomes should be listed on the evaluation tool so students can rate how well they believe they achieved those learning outcomes. Other questions can be included on the course evaluation as well, such as:

- Did faculty clearly make the connection between the course learning outcomes and the concepts that were taught?
- Did the teaching strategies engage you in activities to develop a thorough understanding of the concepts addressed in the course?
- Did the teaching strategies provide ample opportunity to apply concepts to nursing and patient situations in the classroom?
- Did the teaching strategies provide ample opportunity to apply concepts taught in the classroom to nursing and patient situations in the clinical setting?
- Did the evaluation methods used provide a clear understanding of your achievements and learning needs?

Other questions can be asked based on the needs of individual nursing programs. Of major importance is the students' evaluation of whether the course activities provided the opportunity to meet the course learning outcomes and learn the concepts presented in the course. It is imperative that all faculty use concept-based teaching strategies such as those described in this book. Students' evaluation of these teaching strategies is important because it answers two questions:

1. Were the teaching strategies effective from the students' viewpoint?
2. Did the students understand the purpose of the teaching strategies?

Students who value teaching strategies as important to their learning and understand the reasons for the teaching strategies used are more motivated to engage in the learning activities (Cannon & Boswell, 2012). This motivation is as important for clinical education as it is for classroom sessions. Both classroom and clinical experiences in the concept-based curriculum may be very different from students' previous experiences. Focused learning activities used in the clinical experience to enhance students' learning of a concept, such as the example provided for *Collaboration*, may not appear as important to students as spending time performing psychomotor skills. Therefore it is imperative that faculty explain very clearly to students the importance of the activities to the development of their professional identity.

Measuring Faculty Perception of Achievement of Course Learning Outcomes

Faculty evaluation of the curriculum is also elicited (Giddens & Morton, 2010). The frequency of faculty evaluation of the curriculum depends on the evaluation plan established by the nursing program. Faculty complete a survey that asks questions about their involvement in the implementation of the program. It is important to solicit information about the success of teaching strategies, as well as problems encountered. Faculty are invited to provide suggestions based on data to improve the curriculum.

Measuring Program Outcomes

As discussed at the beginning of this chapter, program outcomes are measurable, consumer-oriented indexes designed to evaluate the degree to which the program is achieving its mission and goals. A number of these measures exist. Some of the measures are easy to obtain and provide objective data, such as the first-time pass rate on the National Council Licensure Examination (NCLEX) and the completion rate. The employment rate is also an objective measure but is often difficult to obtain because of lack of contact with graduates. Equally important, but somewhat subjective in nature and often very difficult to obtain, are data related to graduate and employer satisfaction. In this context, satisfaction refers to the belief of the graduate and employer that the curriculum was current and rigorous enough to educate nurses in the delivery of safe, quality, evidence-based care.

NCLEX Pass Rate

While the NCLEX pass rate for prelicensure nursing programs is reported quarterly in most states, the annual pass rate is used as the primary evaluation measure. All state Boards of Nursing and both nursing accreditation bodies require a specific passing rate. However, the required pass rate varies among the state Boards of Nursing. These required pass rate requirements are established because they are viewed as an indication of prelicensure program quality (Spurlock, 2013), and thus the NCLEX pass rate is a critical measure. All prelicensure nursing programs are responsible for providing students with a curriculum that prepares them for the NCLEX. A review of the detailed NCLEX test plan reveals that the bulk of the test plan is based on concepts, and thus a concept-based curriculum is a practical way to prepare graduates.

When analyzing NCLEX pass rates, faculty should consider more than the annual pass rate to determine if the program is providing the education needed for a passing score on the examination. The National Council of State Boards of Nursing makes the NCLEX Program Reports available to nursing programs. The data reported are important because they reflect actual performance on the NCLEX. These reports provide a wealth of information about the scores of the school's students in specific curriculum areas compared with other graduates. These specific areas align with many of the concepts in a concept-based curriculum. For example, the reports include the graduates' achievement in areas such as nutrition; elimination; comfort, rest, activity, and mobility; growth and development; and immunity, as well as many other areas that align with curricular concepts.

These NCLEX Program Reports are published twice a year. Faculty can determine the trend in the data over a number of reporting periods to identify areas that are consistently weak and for which curriculum changes should be considered.

Student Completion Rates

Nursing programs often have highly selective admission requirements and therefore often admit students with higher qualifications than other programs offered by the educational institution. Retaining students so they progress to graduation is a goal of nursing programs for many reasons. Nursing accreditation agencies look at completion rates as one key quality indicator. In the CCNE guidelines, effective in 2014, schools are expected to have a 70% completion rate (CCNE, 2013).

Students should be able to complete the program within the time frame specified in the plan of study and successfully pass the NCLEX, which is the stated goal so students can obtain employment and make use of their education as a practicing professional. Equally important and of primary interest to institutional and nursing accreditation bodies is the students' ability to pay back any school loans. For these reasons, schools have the responsibility to provide a curriculum that is achievable by students who meet the entrance requirements.

As faculty build a concept-based curriculum, they should plan classroom and clinical activities that are achievable. When developing classroom teaching strategies, faculty should expect students to engage in active preparation for class, which may include listening to narrated presentations, completing worksheets, and researching websites in addition to completing assigned readings. Faculty must consider the amount of time an average student needs to complete the class preparation assignments. A general guideline is that for each hour in the classroom, the student can be expected to spend 2 hours outside the classroom engaged in homework. Applying this guideline can help faculty plan assignments without overloading the student, which often leads to the failure of the student to complete the work, thus jeopardizing his or her ability to complete the course requirements. A major advantage of the concept-based curriculum is the elimination of unnecessary content that leads to an oversaturated curriculum and student frustration (Giddens & Brady, 2007). These are major considerations that have an impact on the completion rate, which is an important program outcome measure.

Employment Rate and Employer Satisfaction

Another goal of a quality nursing program is a high rate of employment of the graduates. The employment rate is closely tied to the employer satisfaction rate. When employers are satisfied with graduates of a nursing program, they hire those graduates rather than graduates from programs with lower satisfaction rates. Information about employer satisfaction is often difficult to obtain. The nursing program's Advisory Committee should have representation from employers of the program's graduates. Important roles of the Advisory Committee are to engage in discussion about the performance of graduates and determine the number of graduates hired. Employers are encouraged to be honest and share their opinions of the graduates' performance.

The nursing program Advisory Committee is also a source for input about the concept-based curriculum. Members of the Advisory Committee are stakeholders in the program because they have an interest in the program's graduates as potential employees and/or as clinical students in their facilities. For this reason, it is important to share the structure and basis of the curriculum with these Committee members and request their input about the concepts studied in the program. It may be helpful to list the concepts taught in the program and ask members of the Committee to rate the importance of each concept in their place of employment. This information can be used when faculty review curricular concepts.

Employer satisfaction is also gauged through a formal survey. The survey should ask the employer to rate the new graduate's performance with regard to the behaviors and characteristics that are indicative of the program learning outcomes. These ratings inform the faculty about how well the program learning outcomes are applied in practice. Employers should also be asked to note any job responsibilities the newly hired graduates are expected to perform frequently but that they were not prepared to do. This type of questioning provides information about elements that may be missing in the program.

Graduate Satisfaction

Some accrediting bodies find that graduate satisfaction is an important indicator of a quality program. Typically a survey is sent to graduates between 6 to 9 months after graduation. The same questions included on the employer satisfaction survey can be included on the graduate satisfaction survey but from the perspective of the graduate. That is, graduates should be asked how well they can perform the behaviors and characteristics that are indicative of the program learning outcomes and if they have encountered any job responsibilities they are expected to perform frequently that they were not prepared to do. A difficulty with these surveys is obtaining a high return rate. However, without obtaining information from the employers and the graduates, it is difficult to determine if the concept-based curriculum is preparing graduates for practice.

Summary

Curriculum evaluation is an important and expected process for all schools of nursing. In a concept-based curriculum, it is particularly important that the evaluation methods include assessment of the way the program is being taught. That is, are all faculty engaged in teaching the concept-based curriculum using concept-based teaching strategies? Assessing the implementation of the program is critical to ensure that the students are experiencing a concept-based curriculum.

Program evaluation is particularly important when a new curriculum is implemented (Giddens, 2010). When a new curriculum is implemented, the program outcome of NCLEX pass rates is always a concern. Therefore careful collection and analysis of evaluation data are critical to determine a cause and effect between the new curriculum and program outcomes.

REFERENCES

Accreditation Commission for Education in Nursing: *Standards and criteria*, Atlanta, GA, 2013a, Author.

Accreditation Commission for Education in Nursing: *Glossary*, Atlanta, GA, 2013b, Author.

Cannon S, Boswell C: *Evidence-based teaching in nursing: A foundation for educators*, Sudbury, MA, 2012, Jones & Bartlett.

Caputi L, Blach D: *Teaching nursing using concept maps*, Glen Ellyn, IL, 2008, DuPage Press.

Commission on Collegiate Nursing Education: *Standards for accreditation of baccalaureate and graduate nursing programs*, Washington, DC, 2013, Author.

Davis PE, Grinnell SM, Niemer LM: Laying a foundation for evaluating curricular performance: Tools of the trade, *Journal of Nursing Education* 52(12):671–678, 2013.

Giddens JF, Brady D: Rescuing nursing education from content saturation: A case for a concept-based curriculum, *Journal of nursing education* 46(2):65–69, 2007.

Giddens JF, Morton N: Report card: An evaluation of a concept-based curriculum, *Nursing Education Perspectives* 31(6):372–377, 2010.

Merriam SB, Caffarella RS, Baumgartner LM: *Learning in adulthood: A comprehensive guide*, 3rd ed., San Francisco, CA, 2007, Jossey Bass.

Spurlock D: The promise and peril of high-stakes tests in nursing education, *Journal of Nursing Regulation* 4(1):4–8, 2013.

Appendix A
Clinical Activities Focusing on Concepts

Linda Caputi

The activities in this Appendix are examples of learning that focus students' perceptual awareness on the study of concepts in the clinical setting. The activities provide an in-depth study of a concept. The two students completing the assignment present their work in post-conference. All students learn from that work and are expected to use that learning in the care of patients in a variety of health care settings throughout the nursing program. The thinking required to complete the assignment is of equal importance to the study of the concept.

Concept of Evidence

Activity: Evidence-Based Practice Guidelines

The National Guidelines Clearinghouse (NGC) is a public resource for evidence-based practice guidelines: www.guidelines.gov

Considering your patient for today, visit the NGC website and find one evidence-based practice guideline that applies to the care you will provide today.

Then, identify one other source of evidence-based nursing care that can be applied to your patient.

Respond to the following:
1. Provide a brief explanation of the care you are providing.

2. What guidelines did you investigate?

3. Will you change your approach to care after reading these guidelines? If so, how? If not, why not?

Concept of Patient Education

Activity: Patient Education Related to the Concepts of Development and Culture

1. Identify the discharge and teaching needs of your patient.
2. How will the patient's developmental level (**Concept of Development**), age (**Concept of Development**), and culture (**Concept of Culture**) affect your teaching?
3. Identify who you will teach, their literacy level, and their knowledge base related to the information you will be teaching.
4. Use the following questions to focus your teaching planning.
5. Develop a concept map to explain the factors influencing your teaching of this patient.

Guiding questions:

1. Is patient/family ready to learn?

2. What learning outcomes must occur before the patient/family can be discharged?

3. What are the patient/family's perceived learning needs?

4. Are there barriers to learning (language, literacy, stress, physical distractions)?

5. How does the patient/family wish to have information presented (verbal, written, chart/diagram)?

6. How will you evaluate the learning outcomes?

Concept of Health Care Organizations

Activity: Analyzing the Clinical Microsystem

From the website www.clinicalmicrosystem.org, retrieve the document: The Clinical Microsystem Workbook.

Two students will spend a day completing two tools found in *The Clinical Microsystem Workbook*:

Inpatient Unit Profile

Inpatient Unit Unplanned Activity Tracking Card

Answer these questions:

1. What did you learn about an inpatient unit that you were not aware of?

2. What aspects of the clinical microsystem did you recognize that might lead to nurses making errors?

3. What changes can be made on the unit to prevent errors?

Concept of Health Care Quality

Activity: Nursing-Sensitive Indicators/Quality Improvement Measures

What nursing-sensitive indicators and quality improvement projects are in use on the unit?	What nursing-sensitive indicators and quality measures apply to your patient?	How are the nursing-sensitive quality indicators measured?	What screening tools are used?	What gaps are present in patient care and how will you apply the nursing-sensitive indicators and quality improvement projects to improve patient care?

Concept of Safety

Activity: National Patient Safety Goal Activity

1. Research the Joint Commission's safety initiatives for the hospital and any other environment you will be experiencing in this clinical.
2. Identify ways the healthcare agency addresses these safety goals.
3. Identify ways the agency may improve upon application of each safety goal.

Safety goal:	This agency addresses this goal by:	An improvement might be:

Concept of Collaboration

Activity: Conflict Resolution

Interview a nurse and one other health care provider to identify an area of conflict on the unit	Ask the nurse and health care professional how the conflict was resolved	Observe the interactions of all the health care professionals on the unit	What conflicts did you observe, and how were they handled or not handled?	Analyze the results of your data collection. Explain the effectiveness of the way each conflict was handled and explain how you would have handled the situation differently

Once the above is completed, on subsequent days answer these questions:

Identify a conflict on the unit and how you would resolve it.

Day 1:

Day 2:

Day 3:

Day 4:

Concept of Technology and Informatics

Activity: Analyzing Technology

Type of technology (List all technology used: computer charting, fetal monitors, IV pumps, pulse oximeters, etc.)	How the technology is used	Who accesses the technology	How does the technology contribute to safe, quality care?
Describe how you used the technology	**Discuss your application of the technology to document patient care**		**Discuss your application of the technology to communicate patient information**

Appendix B

Preparing a Concept for Concept-Based Teaching:
Explanation and Template

Beth Rodgers

Cooncept-based teaching requires a change in the traditional teaching model. In order to be effective at concept-based teaching, it is essential to be clear about the concepts that are being taught. Consistency in preparation and approach can be helpful to students as they learn the concepts presented in the curriculum. Thorough preparation in regard to phenomena, concepts, language, related concepts, contexts, and exemplars are critical to the success of teaching concepts.

The steps below can be used to identify phenomena and associated concepts, to ensure the best language and terminology are used, and to help organize ideas for presenting the concept to students. Discussed below is a listing of the components necessary for teaching related to a concept and discussion of each element.

At the end of this material, there is a template that can be used for additional concept clarification. The template can be used along with the components of concept presentation that were addressed in Chapter 6. Once the concept is clearly defined, presentation should include assessment, populations and risk factors, and clinical management, as well as physiologic processes, theoretical links, and other aspects that are appropriate for students to grasp the concept and its application.

Step 1: What Is the Phenomenon?

A phenomenon is an experience as it is perceived by the person having the experience, and a short narrative about the phenomenon can be an excellent starting point. Concepts are used to organize experience, and the experiences that are organized are based on phenomena. For example, the phenomenon of interest for a class session may be how the body regulates temperature or the amount of heat in the body. This phenomenon appears in situations of merely being alive, as a certain temperature or degree of heat is essential for human life. There is more heat when there are inflammatory or infectious processes occurring (and other examples) and heat is reduced when blood vessels dilate to dissipate heat such as in cases of shock. Exposure to cold external temperatures can cause the body to lose heat and make adjustments to maintain the temperature necessary for survival of the brain and organs. This phenomenon is associated with a number of concepts, one of which is *Heat*. If the focus is on how heat is balanced, then the concept might be *Thermoregulation*. If the focus is only on insufficient heat, the concept could be *Hypothermia*. Do not identify the concept at this point; keep the focus on the situation that is of interest.

Step 2: Where Is the Phenomenon Found?

This discussion can be included with the description, above, if that is easier. In some cases, discussion of the situation or cases in which the phenomenon is encountered can be illuminating. For example, is heat associated only with environmental exposure or can it be found in other contexts? Continuing with the example of *Temperature* or *Thermoregulation*, this phenomenon is found in all cases of animal life. In regard to nursing, the phenomenon of thermoregulation can be found in all situations that involve human beings. It is not specific to age, setting, wellness or illness orientation, or other factors. It is inherent in working with humans in any manner. Encourage students to think outside of the typical circumstances as a way to reinforce the understanding of the concept.

Step 3: What Is the Concept and Appropriate Terminology?

After completing the steps above, the appropriate concepts will come into focus for the teaching-learning experience. Keep in mind that the concept is not the same as the word! Identification of the concept needs to involve selection of the appropriate word. Concepts can be expressed using different terminology that sometimes, but not always, conveys the same characteristics. Is there a difference in *Temperature Regulation* and *Thermoregulation*? What is the "best" terminology to use as the focus? Acknowledging other terminology that conveys the same concept can help students avoid confusion and expand their ability to communicate with others.

Step 4: What Other Concepts Are Similar or Related?

No concept exists in a vacuum. A concept is part of a complex network of related ideas, connected in some way, due to similarity, difference, or interdependence. *Thermoregulation*, for example, is related to *Metabolism, Circulation,* and a variety of other concepts. Identifying these connections can help to structure the presentation of a concept to students so they do not view concepts and related phenomena in isolation. In some cases, discussion of similar concepts is essential to clarifying the primary concept of interest. *Grief* and *Bereavement*, for example, sometimes are discussed as interchangeable, yet recognizing the difference in these two concepts is critical to understanding the experience of loss and the associated response. *Sleepiness* and *Fatigue* can easily be confused, yet failure to differentiate which concept is appropriate in a particular situation can result in missed problem identification and ineffective treatment plans.

Step 5: What Are the Key Components (Attributes) of the Concept?

Having selected the concept and the appropriate terminology to express it, the critical process of identifying the key components of the concept can begin. The purpose here is to identify the essential aspects of the concept, specifically the attributes of the concept. This can be done by selecting exemplary cases to analyze, reviewing current and quality literature to analyze discussions of the concept, etc. See Chapter 3: Development of Concepts for Concept-Based Teaching, for more information about components (attributes) of concepts.

Step 6: What Is the Context for an Instance of the Concept?

Context includes a description of the general situation in which an example of the concept is appropriate. In the case of *Thermoregulation*, contexts include infection, exposure, exercise, anything that causes vascular change, certain neurologic conditions as well as maintenance of basal metabolism. The context similarly includes a temporal element, including precipitating events and outcomes. Precipitating events sometimes are part of the context (such as exposure) but also may include antecedents such as medications that cause vasodilation or an increase in activity level. Consequences, or outcomes, of thermoregulation include, if the concept is executed successfully, maintenance of an optimal body temperature. Consequences, or outcomes, may also include results of ineffective regulation such as hypo- or hyperthermia. The thermoregulatory mechanism itself involves physiologic responses such as change in the peripheral vascular system, sweating, and if those are successful, optimal temperature is maintained in the body. This question of context involves a number of facets that are critical to an understanding of the concept.

Step 7: Present Examples

Examples may be developed based on the clinical experience of the instructor, situations the students see in their clinical experience, examples found in the literature or case studies created based on a multitude of sources. Examples should not be thought of as the "model cases," as seen commonly in many approaches to concept analysis. It is important that students be confronted with the wide range of variation in a concept, not merely the ideal or model cases. They will see concepts on a dynamic continuum; encourage students to keep an open mind as knowledge changes and concepts change with that new knowledge. Examples help students learn to apply the concept effectively, but should not be construed or presented in a manner that could place limits on conceptual understanding. The examples that are most appropriate in the teaching-learning situation will vary based on the learning experience and the focus on the conceptual teaching.

Template for Concept Clarification

1. What is the phenomenon?

2. Where is the phenomenon found?

3. What is the concept?

   A. Identify the best term or label for the concept that relates to the phenomenon.

   B. What other terms are used to express the concept? (same idea/concept, but alternate terms)

4. What other concepts are similar or related? Describe differences and similarities.

5. What are the key components (attributes) of the concept?

6. What are common contexts for the concept?

   A. The concept is likely to apply in what situations?

   B. What are precipitating factors or events?

   C. What are outcomes or results?

7. Develop or describe examples. Consider the range of variation and not just ideal examples.

Index

Note: Page numbers followed by f indicate figures; t, tables; b, boxes.

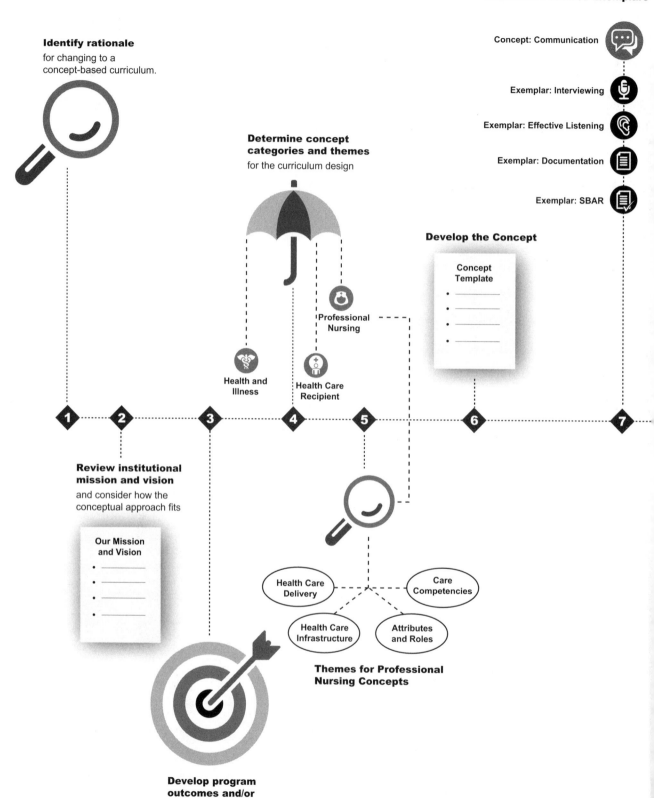

Select the Featured Exemplars

Concept: Communication

Exemplar: Interviewing

Exemplar: Effective Listening

Exemplar: Documentation

Exemplar: SBAR

Identify rationale
for changing to a
concept-based curriculum.

**Determine concept
categories and themes**
for the curriculum design

Develop the Concept

Concept
Template

Professional
Nursing

Health and
Illness

Health Care
Recipient

1 2 3 4 5 6 7

**Review institutional
mission and vision**
and consider how the
conceptual approach fits

Our Mission
and Vision

Health Care
Delivery

Care
Competencies

Health Care
Infrastructure

Attributes
and Roles

**Themes for Professional
Nursing Concepts**

**Develop program
outcomes and/or
competencies**